FROM ORDINARY TO
EXTRAORDINARY
Straight Talk From a Personal Trainer

LAURIE ELLSWORTH

Selah Press
PUBLISHING

From Ordinary To Extraordinary, Straight Talk From a Personal Trainer
By Laurie Ellsworth

Editor: Anna J. Cooke
Managing Editor: Kayla Fioravanti
Water Bottle Image: Vecteezy.com
Copyright © 2018 Laurie Ellsworth

ISBN-13: 978-0692094792 (Selah Press)
ISBN-10: 0692094792

Printed in the United States of America
Published by Selah Press, LLC

Unless otherwise noted, Scripture quotations are taken from The New Living Bible (NLT) Tyndale House Publishers. (2004). Holy Bible: New Living Translation. Wheaton, Ill: Tyndale House Publishers.

Notice of Liability
The author has made every effort possible to check and ensure the accuracy of the information and recipes presented in this book. However, the information herein is sold without warranty, either expressed or implied. The author, publisher, nor any dealer or distributor of this book will be held liable for any damages caused either directly or indirectly by the instructions or information contained in this book.

Disclaimer
Information in this book is NOT intended as medical advice, or for use as diagnosis or treatment of a health problem, or as a substitute for consulting a licensed medical professional. The contents and information in this book are for informational use only and are not intended to be a substitute for professional medical advice, diagnosis, or treatment. Always seek the advice of your physician or other qualified health provider for medical conditions. Never disregard professional medical advice or delay in seeking it because of something you read in this book or any resource.

Dedication

For Mike, my dearest friend in the world and the love of my life.

You've always encouraged me to pursue my dreams but none of them could ever match what I've found in your love.

Acknowledgments

It's been 18 years since my first book, *A Heart of Excellence, How To Succeed At What Matters Most*. There are many reasons for that painful, large gap of time—which I'll probably write about in the next book—but I've known for years that I was supposed to write this second book. Sometimes you just need someone to nudge you forward and get you to start typing on that intimidating and very blank first page. That "someone" was my Heartprint Writer's Group at Grace Chapel. Every single one of you have spoken courage into me and made what was dead come alive again. It has been magnificent and beautiful and hard. (Remember when I couldn't even read the Intro to this book without getting choked up?) I was keenly aware as I was read my rough draft to you that it was your voice—all of your voices—filling the gap of those many silent years with overwhelming kindness and faith in the possibilities of what could be. Whoever underestimates the power of that kind of love has never stared a blank sheet of paper in the face for 18 years and finally won. Because of you, our voices have created a song. And I'm thankful to be in your choir.

Lona Fraser, our fearless leader, you champion all of our ideas and give them wings to morph from simple, abstract ideas into proliferation of the written word. There is simply no one like you. Your joy is contagious and godly and beautiful.

Thank you to my publisher and mentor, Kayla Fioravanti with Selah Publishing, who literally had the patience of Job waiting for me to finish each round of changes. Your kindness has fueled my confidence for these 3 years and I thank you from the bottom of my heart.

Thank you to Donna Rose whose faithful friendship for over 30 years has been a healing balm and light in my life. As the first reader, (was it really 3 years ago that I finished it for the first time?), you were encouraging in every way when I was ready to shuck it and start over.

Thank you to each of my grown children: David, Allie, and Evan. I have learned so much from each of you about working hard and finishing strong, no matter the cost. What you have already accomplished in your lives is so inspiring to me, and I'm over-the-moon grateful that I get to be your mom.

Thank you to my Food Scientist, daughter-in-love, Jessica Spanton, who first taught me about gut health and that healthy food can taste awesome, even Kombucha.

Thank you to my Plexus tribe with whom I share the incredible responsibility and honor of helping others find true health solutions that are life-changing.

Thank you to every friend that has ever prayed over me. You mean the world to me and I've been so blessed to walk this journey with you, some of the most incredible people in the world.

Lastly, thank you to my husband, Mike Ellsworth, who stayed committed to this book and its message of courage when I let doubt creep in and delay its completion. You are a Knight in shining armor and I could fill the world with all of your good deeds and thoughtful acts of kindness. How did I ever get so lucky? xo

Contents

Introduction... 1

Chapter 1   Liquid Gold... 7

Chapter 2   Drink Like a Fish... 19

Chapter 3   Sleep Like a Baby... 27

Chapter 4   Sweet Dreams are Made of These..................... 39

Chapter 5   Get Movin'!... 57

Chapter 6   Do What You Love—It Will Love You Back 77

Chapter 7   Food Is Fuel... 89

Chapter 8   Fuel Your Body...For Real...With REAL Food...... 107

Reach Laurie... 125

Decide, Plan & Begin... 127

Plan Tomorrow Beginning Today..................... 133

Contract of Commitment......................... 135

I AM... 137

Grocery List... 139

Recipes... 145

Eating Out... 147

Healthy Habit Checklist......................... 149

Health Habit Journal......................... 151

Book Recommendations......................... 213

Bibliography... 215

Introduction

At the tender age of 23, I endured a heart-breaking divorce after only 4 years of marriage. Our beautiful son, David, was only 3-years-old at the time. It was crushing. I'd always dreamed, as every little girls does, that my marriage would be made in heaven and last forever. When it fell apart, I found myself completely and utterly devastated. Suffice it to say, a very significant part of me died and I wondered if I would ever be whole again. I turned to food for comfort—lots of comfort—which only led to more anguish and guilt. It became a miserable cycle of self-defeat, despair, and lonliness.

As so often happens, that emotional brokenness manifested itself physically and I ended up gaining 35 pounds in 6 months! I went from a size 5 to a 15! And then tried everything possible to lose the weight, from the crazy to the scary. I turned to every diet gimmick available and lived on a constant binge-starvation cycle. I couldn't sleep. My hair fell out in clumps. My stomach was in a constant state of nausea. My cycle stopped completely. I felt a very heavy sense of embarrassment every time I looked in the mirror. I was falling apart inside and it became impossible to hide it on the outside. People tend to notice when you gain that much weight and patches of your hair fall out. Fatigue was my constant companion and yet I struggled to sleep. I felt exhausted, overwhelmed, and hopeless pretty much every day.

I had grown up in a Christian home and loved Jesus from childhood. But thirty-eight years ago, divorce was a Scarlet letter. There were no support groups or Grief Share or Celebrate Recovery. Only finger shaking and looks of "good girls don't get divorced." I tried to fight through the shame but it got the best of me. I had a difficult time even going to church. I believed the lie that God couldn't possibly still love me. I'd strayed too far. Failed with the sacred. Fallen too many times. Too dirty to lift my hands.

But love pursued me through a group of strong, mercy-filled women who reached out to me with incredible kindness. No hurtful comments about weight gain or missing pieces of hair. These women were for real and they were prepared to do battle on my behalf. They were fervently praying for me, and I mean on-your-knees-crying-out-for-help kind of prayer. You know, the kind of prayer that Jesus would've prayed—one of compassion, forgiveness, and hope.

As those women opened their arms and hearts to me, I slowly began to lift my head. I very nervously attended church for the first time in a long time, sitting in the back row as I recall. But as I quietly dared to join in worship, I began to find a new voice inside of me. Timid at first, but the more I sang the more I felt a tender wave of peace rush over me. It was the song of grace welcoming me back. It was the love of a father yearning to hold his lost child.

Worship has a way of gripping your heart in a way that touches and cleanses every part of your soul. It's a powerful weapon against darkness. It binds up emotional wounds as you start to tangibly feel how wide, how deep, how long, and how high the love of God really is for you. It's the sweet song that chases into hidden places to rescue those sinking in the mud and mire. And I was drowning in the stuff.

As new habits formed, the extra weight began to fall off, I began to heal physically, and I started to feel a deep transformation in my soul that was making me new from the inside out. I physically felt more alive than I had in years!

There were new spiritual habits that also helped me wipe the slate clean and begin afresh. I realized I had been going about faith all wrong. I thought I had to earn God's love by being slightly better than I was sinful. Balancing the scales, so to speak, in favor of good deeds. And certainly never committing a *big* sin like divorce.

But grace redeemed it ALL. Healed it ALL. And brought miracles into my life that gave me a brand new song to sing! Restoration flooded my soul and gave me the courage I needed to get up and try again. And I didn't do it alone.

I met a wonderful man about this time who thought I was the coolest thing since sliced bread. This was a miracle in and of itself because as you now know—I was quite messed up. We married a year after we met and just celebrated 33 years!

Day by day, the shackles came off.

Powerfully compelled to help others avoid the same excruciating mistakes I had made, I stepped forward into a higher calling. Health education became my new language.

Since I was my own first client, it was a valuable internship for my future personal training. I had tried every ridiculous fad there was, knew every excuse in the book, and had been quite successful at sabotaging any good habits that had been conceived in a moment of sober discipline. Yep, I knew all the excuses that seem rationale at the time but only kept me defeated.

Never one to just stick a big toe in the water and test it gradually, I totally immersed myself into this new calling by going back to school to get a degree in Kinesiology from the *University of Illinois*. I taught college health and fitness classes for 15 years and worked as a personal trainer and life coach for over 25 years, pouring into others and helping them find their own new level of extraordinary success. In 2000, I wrote my first book, *A Heart of Excellence: How to Succeed at What Matters Most*, and starting speaking at conferences around the country.

So, here's the thing. I know firsthand what it feels like to be stuck in an awful and debilitating emotional prison. And I know what it's like to use a counterfeit anesthesia to soothe yourself. I've walked in those well-worn shoes that temporarily mask the pain but only make things worse. I've also walked with thousands of clients that have struggled in their own difficult journey. So trust me when I say, if you've got issues you're not alone. There may be people that have never struggled mightily—I've just never met any. And I'm old. So I'm thinking they probably don't exist.

Everyone, and I mean everyone, wants to feel better in some way.

They want to feel like they have risen above "ordinary" and are living at an extraordinary level! But life is hard and stress is real to the point it can feel like a beat down at the end of the day. So people look for relief or comfort. The problem is that relief and comfort from the wrong places only bring more desperation, regret, and pain. And that struggle often makes us feel that other important aspirations are out of reach as well. Like a good night's sleep. Like a body that doesn't ache every time we move. Like losing weight for good. Like accomplishing professional goals and career advancements. Like writing a book from ideas that have been swirling in your head for years and maybe even decades. Like hopes and dreams for an extraordinary future.

As one who was dying in the valley and now lives most days on a mountaintop, I can tell you there is a much better way to live. And it starts with a beautiful and intentional journey to a better, stronger YOU! As you grow and step forward with courage, you'll begin to master a few new habits. Then a few more. Then, the small changes become BIG changes. Before you know it, the ordinary is no more. You will feel and be EXTRAORDINARY!

George Burns quipped at his 90th birthday party, "If I had known I was going to live so long, I would have taken better care of myself." We all would, wouldn't we?! And as long as we're still breathing we can. A few new habits at a time. Over time. For a lifetime. That's how you get there.

So that's the kind of book you're reading—written by someone whose past has been marked by   but now lives a transformed life that is exploding with abundant energy, overwhelming peace, and mountain-moving faith. Extraordinarily new.

Love did that. Grace rescued me. Truth instructed me. Simple tools I now share with you. For YOUR extraordinary journey of courage and renewal. You got this, friend. You really do.

"Do not despise these small beginnings
for the Lord rejoices to see the work begin."
Zechariah 4: 10

This book is a compilation of real-life conversations with hundreds of personal training clients, portrayed through one fictitious client named Emily. (hSo, if I've ever trained you, that means it's not you!) The interactions depicted in this book with Emily are through my lens as a personal trainer and life coach. They capture the good, the bad, and the ugly moments we all face as we move out of our comfort zone into a higher level of living.

As a fly on the wall during personal training sessions, you'll garner an inside perspective of the struggles and victories that mark the courageous lives of those who dare to attempt, and ultimately accomplish, remarkable and lasting change. In their health. In their energy. In their faith. In their peace. In their dreams. And in the final result, their ability to believe that anything is possible with God.

Chapter 1
Liquid Gold

"Hey, good morning!" I greeted Emily enthusiastically. "It's so wonderful to meet you. Welcome to our community!"

Emily, my new personal training client, had just moved to the area to work as a Senior Vice President of a large marketing company.

Unfortunately, Emily seemed a little less charged to see me. I settled for a head nod and a muffled, "Mornin'."

Okey dokey. Not everyone is a morning person. No worries.

"Before we jump in, Emily, as I look over your profile it says under "remarks" that you have some questions for me. How may I help you?" I asked, eagerly.

"I just want to know one thing," Emily began, immediately cutting to the chase.

"Sure, fire away."

"How in the world can I stop feeling like crap, lose some weight, and get some flippin' energy?"

Well alrighty then. No beating around the bush for this lady.

"I'm glad you asked, Emily." That's exactly what I specialize in—helping people make simple, yet powerful changes in their health so they can feel amazing and energized all through the day! And of course that colors every part of your life, so it is incredibly important. I have some tools to share with you that I know will make a tremendous difference for you."

"Good! I'm glad to hear that. Because, honestly, I've lost count of the number of programs I've tried. And I have yet to find one that delivers any kind of "amazing" results," Emily said, using air quotes. "I'm so tired of programs that over-promise and under-deliver. I'm really needing this one to be different. Know what I mean?"

Boy, do I, sweet sister! I know EXACTLY what you mean! How many gazillion times did I get my hopes up as I started a new weight loss plan that THIS time would be different—that I would actually make progress on getting my life and health back on track without some crazy cockamamie scheme! Oh honey, do I ever know the heartache of so many disappointing attempts!! This is exactly why you are standing here in front of me, ready to try just one more time. God arranged for you to be with a trainer that has been where you are. So, my dear friend, you have come to the right place. I definitely know what you mean, Em.

I reassured Emily as I kept my emotions in check that I understood completely. "This program *is* different, Emily. What sets it apart is that it's sustainable and not something you go on and off of. These are habits, tools, and changes that can help you for the rest of your life! Everything I'm going to teach you is what I used to rise out of the funk I was in and take charge of my life. It helped me break free from the seemingly "normal" habits like diet soda, skipping meals, and yo-yo dieting that kept stealing my progress. It helped me transform my heart and head so I could lose weight and NEVER gain it back! I learned a new way to live that has given me explosive energy and freed me from my sugar cravings and food additions. It helped me conquer my self-doubt and gave me a renewed confidence to pursue dreams that once seemed impossible. Now I feel more alive than ever and that's exactly what I expect for you, Emily!"

Emily was a bit stunned with my confident declarations but then finally nodded approvingly and said "Well, alright! Wow! I like the sound of that!"

"Over the next few weeks, you'll be writing, recording, and planning like never before to help you eliminate old habits by developing new ones. We want to make sure the changes and improvements you make are not just short-term, but ones that you keep forever and ever. And one of the best ways to ensure that is to write them down. What good is making changes that rock your world if you can't keep them, you know?"

"Right! I need good habits to stick like crazy glue. You ever get that on a finger? Man, now THAT lasts forever!"

Laughing, I nodded my head and agreed. "Perfect analogy, Emily. Alright, let's jump right in and start our discussion on how you can start feeling better right away. Today's energy secret is a tool that is going to completely revolutionize your life!"

"Fantastic!"

"I guarantee you it will be one of the most important keys to improve how you feel throughout the day," I said, building the suspense.

"That's what I'm talkin' about!" Emily responded enthusiastically, as though I was about to give her the secret to winning the lottery.

"It's something that can literally change your life. I know it changed mine. It's simple, yet completely remarkable in its power to help you feel better. It's not overstating it to say you can't live without it!"

"Yes! Yes! Yes! Bring it on. Tell me, tell me. What is it?" Emily prodded.

"It's water!!" I exclaimed. "Good ole' fashioned H2O is liquid gold to your body and you are going to start drinking the right amount every day without fail. That's the secret!"

Wha. Wha. Crickets.

Emily was not impressed. "Water? Seriously? I've heard that about a million times so, one, I don't think it's a secret. And two, the only change I see when I drink more water is that I'm up all night peeing. I gotta be honest, that doesn't sound remarkable, powerful or life-changing in any way."

Undaunted, I continued. "You're right, it's not *really* a secret in that most people *know* they should be drinking more water. However, actually doing it is quite another issue. Drinking enough water—and the right amount is usually way more than people think—has immeasurable benefits that can influence energy, digestion, the ability to lose weight, increase concentration, and can drastically improve and, yes, even change lives."

I could see Emily was still skeptical and needed more convincing.

Challenging me, she replied, "Explain how that is possible."

"Emily, too many people are looking for that magic pill that will instantly make them feel better. I know I certainly was. We all want the quick and easy way to immediately feel better and stop the drag that we keeps us from our best. Unfortunately, most people miss out on the incredible benefits of water simply because it seems too easy and they don't understand how significant and essential it is to feeling better. It's true what we constantly hear, Emily. We do need a *lot* more water and here's why: It's the most important nutrient in our bodies! We would literally die without it in a matter of days. I'd say that makes it an enormous priority, wouldn't you?"

I was building my case. Of course anything that keeps us alive should be a top priority! How can anyone argue with that?

"Yes, I would have to say that's probably true," Emily admitted.

"It's impossible to have extreme energy without drinking enough water! Not that it gives us energy directly—that's the job of our food, mainly carbohydrates and fats. But water is the primary component of our blood, every muscle, every organ including our brain, heart, and skin, and all soft tissue. Without it our hearts can't beat and our brains can't function. It enables the completion of all the jobs inside of your body. Every single one. That's why it gives you energy and life."

Emily raised one eyebrow, still not completely persuaded by my dramatic claims but I knew she would come around. The research is just too convincing not to.

I knew it was important to speak Emily's language to help her understand just how important this habit was in making her feel better, so I appealed to her professional role as a Senior VP. "Emily, what would happen to your company and your 500 employees if your electricity was accidentally shut off for an entire day and you had no generator to back it up?" I asked.

"Everyone would panic, including me! It would be a major crisis! It would be impossible to conduct business without the electricity to run our server which runs our intranet and everything else! We would lose all access to the information that runs our show which would make us miss important deadlines! Bottom line is we would lose a lot of money! We simply could not perform at all!"

"That's water, Emily—it's like electricity!" I exclaimed. "Water is a conduit, a life-giving tool through which everything else happens. Without it, nothing works right. We simply can't function! But with it, let me tell you, it's amazing what can be accomplished.

"Here's a list of some of the amazing jobs it helps perform."

- Digestion—water is the vehicle digestion uses to flush waste from our bodies through the liver. It also quickens the time it takes us to poop, which helps prevent colon cancer. As a matter of fact, elimination should be so quick you don't have time to read in the bathroom. Forget about catching up on your favorite magazines, books, or newspapers in there. You want elimination to be quick, easy, and complete. Water is a natural laxative that speeds up this process and has no side effects. And, yes, we're already talking about poop.

- Muscle function—water is essential for building and maintaining proper muscle tone. 80% of our muscle mass is water! Water enables muscles to work all day long for recreation, fun, exercise, and chores.

- Clean kidneys—water helps the kidneys and urinary tract eliminate waste through peeing, which also helps prevent urinary tract infections.

- Fluid regulation—water helps prevent retention and bloating by keeping a healthy flow of fluids on a regular basis. It primes the pump, so to speak, and is a natural diuretic which is the best way to keep all fluids at healthy levels.

- Appetite satiation—water helps us feel full faster so we don't overeat and we don't falsely think we are hungry when we are really just thirsty.

- Fat metabolism—water equips the liver do its job of breaking down fat (both from stored fat and fatty foods) to be used as energy. If you want to lose weight efficiently, water is your best friend.

- Brain function—water enables our brains to maintain concentration and memory so we can focus clearly, whether solving complex analytical problems, balancing our checkbook, or listening to a conversation. Did you know your brain cells can shrink while they're dehydrated? I don't know about you but I need my brain cells working for me, not adding to my brain fog.

- Regulating body temperature—water is responsible for maintaining a healthy temperature around 98.6 degrees. We sweat when we need to cool off and sweat is made from water.

- Lubricating joints—water is the main ingredient in synovial fluid. This is valuable lubricant for your joints, keeping them running smoothly like WD-40 on a squeaky hinge.

- Lubrication for skin, eyes, and lips—water supplies fluid to enhance daily healing and proper moisture levels to these sensitive tissues to help them feel and look their very best. If you're constantly reaching for lip balm, it's an inside hydration issue.

- Protecting organs—water forms a soft barrier around vital organs which protects them during a fall and also enables them to perform their roles flawlessly.

- Dissolving minerals and nutrients—water assists in absorbing and sending nutrients from our food and vitamins to the rest of the body. This helps protect us from nutrient deficiency which can cause diseases in the body.

- Keeps blood thin—water supplies the fluid to keep our blood thin so it can have the right viscosity level. Healthy blood should not be thick and sticky. You want your blood to be thin enough to easily move through the blood vessels without friction or being slowed down."

"So, that's a short list of some of the jobs water performs. Pretty impressive, wouldn't you say?"

"That's the *short* list?" Emily asked, incredulously. "I had no idea water played such a key role in those areas. Okay," Emily admitted reluctantly, "you may be on to something here. How do I know how much water I need through the day?"

"One easy way to calculate a good amount is to take how much you weigh, divide that number in half, then drink that in ounces. For example, if someone weighs 150 pounds, half of that is 75. That person needs about 75 ounces of water each day.

"*The Institute of Medicine* (IOM) continues to recommend 8-13 glasses of water each day for men (8 ounces each), and 8-9 glasses for women[1], but states that most people consume far below that amount. Unfortunately it's not a habit for most of us. But if you ask most people how much water they drink through the day, surprisingly, they believe they are drinking the recommended amount!

"As a personal trainer, I see this time and time again. Most clients, with a few exceptions, confidently estimate they drink enough water—until they actually track their consumption for a few days. About 98% of my clients have been very surprised to discover that they drank only about *half* of what was needed. And of course, if you combine that with copious amounts of diuretics through caffeinated drinks (coffee, tea, soda) and also alcoholic drinks, there is an even greater water loss."

No judgment from this girl...I love a warm, toasty latte in the morning and a relaxing Pinot every so often in the evening. You just have to counter it with extra water so it doesn't exacerbate the problem.

"Hmmm," Emily pondered as she remembered a similar response. "That's exactly what I answered on *my* health questionnaire. I estimated that I drink plenty of water but now I'm not so sure."

"That's okay," I assured her. "What's important is how you move forward. I think you understand now why you have to be so vigilant."

"Yep, I'm getting it. Water is a big deal and it sounds like it can make or break how I feel. Who knew?"

"Well, great and I'm only half done with my spiel," I responded smiling. "We still need to discuss measurement and consequences."

"Measurement and consequences?"

"It's impossible to measure how much water we lose each day because we are constantly using and losing it through sweat, urine, tears, and invisible ways like respiration every time we breathe."

"Yeah, I guess it would be difficult to measure those things."

"Exactly. So what happens if we don't get enough water? Won't we know if we're dehydrated and isn't that why we get thirsty in the first place?"

Emily jumped in. "That's what I was just asking myself! Thirst tells us when we're low, right?"

"Yes, but God designed the thirst mechanism to act like a circuit breaker to tell us when we're *already* at a significant deficit. If we feel thirsty, we already have a shortage."

"Wow, our thirst acts as a protective mechanism? That was a brilliant design."

"Sure was! But it's better to *never* be thirsty—that way you know you've got enough in you.

"Did you know our military has researched this? Tests conducted by the U.S. Army in cold weather show that if soldiers drink only when they are thirsty, they stay in a continuously dehydrated state. So, we actually need to drink water *before* we're thirsty to help us avoid a deficit or we will suffer consequences, which in severe cases can lead to death.

"*Mayo Clinic* states that a lack of water can lead to a state of dehydration, a condition that occurs when you don't have enough water in your body to carry out normal functions. Even a mild form can drain your energy and make you tired.[2] And while there are many levels of dehydration from mild to severe, they all come with unwanted consequences."

"Let's hear about these consequences 'cus I'm pretty sure this will apply to me." Emily confessed.

"The number 1 consequence will come as no surprise—fatigue!"

Emily groaned, "Just what I need!"

"I know, right? Who wants to be exhausted through the day? No one I know! But fatigue is often one of the first symptoms people notice. That means a large percentage of our population is walking around exhausted, dragging themselves through the day, never dreaming their constant tiredness could possibly be from a water shortage. And I know what you're going to say, 'That's not why I'm tired! I'm tired because I don't get enough sleep!'"

"True, very true." Emily interjected.

"While true sleep deprivation obviously causes fatigue, as well as perhaps the side-effect of a prescribed medication or an illness, we are aware when those indicators are present. Outside of those factors, a shortage of water can be the culprit when we feel depleted or run down. Researchers from the *University of Connecticut's Human Performance Laboratory* found that even mild dehydration can cause fatigue.[3] Most of us don't closely correlate those two at all."

"I sure wouldn't."

"And yet, Emily, Even the Bible confirms that drinking enough water will make you look and feel better. In Daniel 1:12-15 it says, 'Give us vegetables and water and see if we don't look better than the others.' And after 10 days of that, Daniel and his 3 friends looked noticeably better and healthier over the others who didn't drink water and eat veggies!"

"Wow, pulling out the big guns, eh?"

I smiled and answered confidently, "You know, I love truth. No one could deny that Daniel and his friends definitely looked better from drinking water and eating vegetables."

"Well I can't argue with that. Point made."

"Here's the rest of the consequences and you may find some of them quite surprising."

"Okay, lay it on me."

"You're sure you ready for this one?"

"Yes! Come on already!"

"Okay, you asked for it. It's *hunger.*"

"No way!" Emily protested.

"Yep! When we're low on water our brains can actually stimulate our appetites since we do get some water from food—up to 20% of our daily need. Looking back on my battle, I can now see how there were many times when I was eating because I was thirsty, not hungry."

"Ugh, I need my appetite stimulated like a hole in the head," Emily grumbled.

"Headaches can be another consequence—*Consumer Reports,* April 28, 2016 states that dehydration may cause a headache, but can often be relieved by simply drinking several ounces of water.[4]

"Also, achy joints can come from dehydration. And doesn't that affect everything you do? When joints hurt, it seems like everything hurts!

I had Emily's rapt attention so I tackled unpleasant digestive issues. "Trouble with pooping, constipation, and hemorrhoids—enough said there?" I asked.

"No need to elaborate."

"Dry skin, dry scalp, dry eyes and lips are common consequences. So often people try to treat these symptoms with expensive hair, skin, and lip products, when in fact we can eliminate the cause of the dryness by..."

"...drinking more water?" Emily interjected.

"You got it, Emily! I know for me, dry lips are one of my first indicators that I need to drink up. Once I get some water in me, my lips respond almost immediately.

"Dehydration can also affect our memory and attention. According to Dr. Laura DeFina, President and Chief Executive Officer of *The Cooper Institute*, brain function interruptions most likely affected by dehydration are short term memory and attention. Dr. DeFina's research shows that in extreme cases, it isn't uncommon to see a marathon runner complete the race, only to receive medical treatment after becoming confused and disoriented.[5] It's is pretty clear that water affects the brain and its intellectual and mental function."

Emily shook her head. "Good night, nurse! Is there anything not affected by water? I mean, no wonder I feel so awful!"

"Not fun stuff, is it? That's why I know you'd rather be drinking enough water and preventing all this stuff! When you conquer this new tool you won't have to deal with these consequences. And won't that feel incredible?"

Emily agreed. "I guess I have just gotten so used to feeling bad that it seems normal." Then she paused and added, "But let's be real here for a minute. You make some solid points and valid arguments but that is a *lot* of water. I'm just being honest here. Isn't there a smaller amount I can drink so I'm not running to the bathroom every 30 minutes?"

"The short answer is no," I said directly. "The long answer is that depends entirely on how many consequences you want. How many side effects of dehydration are you willing to put up with?"

"Well, ideally, none!"

"If you don't want any consequences, then half your body weight in ounces is still your answer for how much you need. And," I added, "Going to the bathroom several times during the day is very healthy. I know it's inconvenient but do you want convenience or health?"

Emily smiled and answered, "I'd like health to be convenient."

"I know. I would too, Emily. But since we know that only peeing a couple of times a day is *not* healthy and can cause terrible side-effects, and drinking enough water can prevent all those, doesn't that alone make 'inconvenience' a little more convenient?

"And you want to lose weight, right? You've got a greater chance of accomplishing that if you drink enough water. It's a tool that can greatly help you reach a lot of your goals. But the choice is yours of course."

Compliance with any habit is only sustainable with ownership and commitment. Emily had to want to feel better more than she wanted to stay with the comfort of her old habits and familiar routine. Drinking more water, as simple as it is, had to be her choice. She had to value it in her own heart and head to keep doing it every day. And over time, what we do every day actually has the biggest impact on our lives.

I could see the wheels turning and the intellectual argument going on in Emily's head. "All right, fine! I do want to get more energy, lose weight more easily and all that other "amazing" jazz. And I know this is a tool that can really help me," she admitted. "Now, just tell me how to stay out of the bathroom all day!"

I lit up and responded, "That, my friend, is our next discussion.

Chapter 2
Drink Like a Fish

After a quick water break, we continued our conversation on Emily's first new tool. We had to get past her objections and fear of being in the bathroom all day. Pronto.

"That is the number one complaint I hear from clients about drinking more water. They have to go to the bathroom so much more often and it's a pain in the neck. So let's discuss that. Does it mean you're drinking *too much* water? Should you *always* pee that often? What happens when you reach the proper hydration level?"

Emily stood with her hands on her hips, raised one eyebrow and said, "Yes, I'd really like to know the answers to all those."

"To begin with," I responded, "our brains are very smart. They are constantly monitoring and regulating our fluid supply, as well as many other things. When we don't drink enough water, our brain senses there is a deficit and immediately starts to hold onto the water we do have through the process of retention. That's why we don't pee as much. But remember, that's a sign of trouble," I reminded Emily.

"Normally in the first few days of drinking more water, you *will* pee more because it's like priming the pump on a well. Your body finally has enough water coming in so it can let go of the water it was holding. Your brain senses an adequate flow of water inside of you so it stops restricting the flow out of your body, and you pee more. After those first few days of letting go of the retained water, peeing should level out but you should still need to go more than 2 or 3 times a day. Actually it's healthy to pee around 5-6 times a day! You'll get used to it!"

"If you say so. I guess it makes sense to me that our brains are working to make sure we keep enough water inside of us. And when there isn't enough, we hang on to the water we do have."

"Exactly, Emily. Now let's discuss how to make this new tool stick. Remember, the right amount of water is one of the crucial foundations to help you *stop feeling like crap, lose weight, and have more energy* which is what you said you wanted. So, are you ready to do this, Emily? Change your hydration and drink like a fish?"

"Woah, I can drink like a fish on this plan??"

"Yes—as long as you drink what a fish drinks," I said jokingly.

"Ah, I knew there was a catch. I can admit that I probably need more water. I can even admit that I have a few of the dehydration consequences from that list that you gave earlier. I'm just not sure how to make it work for me. I mean, I've tried this before and I'm very disciplined for a week or so but then I fall off the wagon and go back to my old ways. And what about the articles I'm reading now that say *all* the liquids you drink, including coffee, count towards your total intake? Can't I just drink coffee to get my water?"

My knee-jerk reaction always tempts me to say *No, coffee does not count because it's a diuretic!* But I've learned over the years it's more powerful when a client comes to that realization through their own critical thinking. It helps them take control of their future behavior because they have worked through the rationale in their own head. It makes more sense to them. And that helps them adopt a new behavior into their lifestyle. And keep it.

"First, Emily, you could always try it out and see if you feel different. Take a few weeks to get used to how you feel when you drink straight water for your hydration. Then test how just coffee makes you feel. What do you think? See if there is a noticeable change and then you will know for sure. You decide.

"Secondly, almost everyone has attempted to start some kind of healthy habit with limited success. For whatever reason, they give up too soon. They may start off strong when motivation and hopes are high, but then get sidetracked from the busyness of life. When they don't notice much change in how they look or feel, momentum fizzles until it's gone completely and they're back to square one. It's a very common obstacle but there are definitely steps you can implement to make this tool work for you, not just for a day or a week, but for a lifetime."

"Well, alrighty then. Let's get going," Emily prodded.

"Before we go over the steps," I cautioned, "I need to have you check your urine every day."

"I have to track how much I pee?" Emily asked, incredulously.

"I want you to check the *color* of your urine, not the quantity," I responded reassuringly. "That's a quick way to measure whether you have an adequate supply of water in your body. The color should be so light it's almost indistinguishable. That lets you know your water intake is properly diluting the impurities in your kidneys and bladder. If it is dark or cloudy then that is a sign you're dehydrated. The color can change through the day depending on your intake and activity level so I want you to monitor it every time you pee. It will take you less than 2 seconds. Okay?" I looked at Emily, waiting for her confirmation.

"Yeah...okay," she agreed.

"Okay, Emily, there are 3 strategies I want to teach you that will really help you sustain your water-drinking habit after the initial inspiration wears off. Which it will, so you may as well plan for it.

"And you can start doing these 3 things right out of the gate to start feeling better immediately."

"Immediately? I like the sound of that."

"Just a forewarning—this is not rocket science and none of these habits are complex or difficult. They are simple and *simple* is the key to getting it done. They do, however, require intentional planning and follow through until they become an automatic habit which can take 3 weeks or longer."

"All right," Emily replied, with just a hint of anticipation. "Three things. I can do that."

"You absolutely can do this, Emily! I have great confidence in you."

Emily smiled, "Okay, ready."

"Number 1: Drink 8-12 ounces of water as soon as you get up in the morning. This is, of course, before any coffee," I added.

"Kill-joy," Emily muttered, winking.

"Keep a glass on your kitchen counter—I keep mine right by the coffee pot—and guzzle a glass of water as soon as your eyes are open. This is also when I take my plant-based digestive enzyme supplements—on an empty stomach. Start your hydration right out of the gate in the morning. It's a powerful start to your day! You're not just drinking water."

"I'm not?" Emily asked, a bit confused.

"No, you're not. You're starting the day with a win! You're establishing a healthy precedent to start the day strong and that is incentive and motivation to continue good choices and habits throughout the entire day!

"I've noticed the way in which we start our day has a significant impact on the good decisions we make all day long. Unfortunately the opposite is true as well. When we don't start strong in the morning, we can tend to make unhealthy choices throughout the day. We've all had days where the morning doesn't start off with committed resolve. We hit the snooze, we're running late, we skip water, breakfast, and a peace-filled morning. Then we compensate through the rest of the day with comfort foods and drinks that only make us feel worse. It is a weak, conscious decision that forms other weak, sub-conscious decisions *all day long*."

"Ouch. That one kind of stings." Emily admitted. "But it makes sense too."

"If you start the day strong with an empowering decision right out of bed, you will tend to make decisions all through the day that agree with it. Momentum perpetuates momentum! If you feel like a winner in the very first moment of the day, there's a greater chance you will feel like a winner through the rest of the day and you'll automatically make decisions that align with that thought."

"I like that—no, I *love* that!" Emily said, surprising both of us with her enthusiasm. "Healthy choices in the morning help me make other good choices throughout the day. I've noticed this does actually happen, but usually the opposite way. I grab a donut or 2 on my way to work and the rest of the day I reach for cookies and caffeine instead of anything good for me. And really, how easy is a glass of water right before coffee or breakfast?!"

"*Very* easy.

"Sounds like you're ready for the second strategy, Em!"

"Absolutely! You're right. Simple is the way to go."

"Number 2: Choose a water bottle to keep with you throughout the day and keep refilling it. We have to make water drinking convenient. Choosing a bottle that stays with you all day is proactively providing a convenient way to drink water. This is really about starting a new rhythm for your day that will make a huge impact on your energy and everything else in your life."

"That's why I'm doing this program—I am just so tired of being tired. A new rhythm sounds like just the ticket I need. So tell me more about these water bottles. What size do I need?"

"I use a bottle that fits into the cup-holder of both my car and the elliptical machines where I work out. It needs to be a convenient size for how you handle it and should be made from material that is BPA-free (Bisphenol A). Measure how much water your bottle holds so you can easily track how much you are consuming each day. Don't leave the house without filling that puppy to the brim. Chug or sip at every stoplight."

"What about bottled water?" Emily asked. "Is that a good option?"

"Bottled spring water can be a convenient option. So a little research on brands so you choose one that you're comfortable with. Just remember, you should *never* refill a plastic bottle that is not BPA free. I really prefer a glass or stainless steel container so I can easily refill it."

"Noted. Buy a good water bottle that is BPA-free, preferably glass or stainless steel. Do you have a favorite brand? I've shopped for them before and it seems like there are hundreds to choose from."

"I personally like Yeti since they keep the water cold and it fits the drink holder in my car. The important thing is that you keep it with you every day and refill it all day long. Easy-peasy."

"You're right. Fairly easy so far. Drink water first thing in the morning and have a bottle ready to go with me through the day. Check and check."

"Let's test your memory, Emily. Do you remember how much water you need in a day?"

"The Institute of Medicine suggests that I drink between 8 and 9 glasses each day, with 8 ounces in each," she quickly responded. "And around 13 glasses a day for men," she added confidently.

"Excellent! Way to go, Emily!"

"Or I can drink half my body weight in ounces!"

"Wow! Emily, I'm so impressed!

"Okay, we're almost done. Our third strategy requires a little more planning," I cautioned, "but it's just as important to your success as the first two."

Emily nodded as she gave me a thumbs up.

"**Number 3: Plan *when* you will drink water.**

"You mean like a schedule?" Emily asked, a bit perplexed.

"I know that sounds a little odd," I admitted, "but we plan important meetings, appointments, and vacations. So why not water? By scheduling it, it's almost a guarantee you will do it! I know it sounds like something maybe only elite athletes do."

"Or crazy people," Emily added, using her finger to make a circle around her ear and then pointed to me.

"I'm not crazy," I laughed. "I've just learned the hard way that I'm forgetful! And apparently I'm not the only one. This is the step where I see most people struggle. They start out with admirable intentions and drink water consistently in the beginning of their program because they're determined and excited. But because they have not consciously planned *when* to drink through the day, they end up quickly forgetting about it when the day gets busy. The excitement wears off and they revert back to their old habits which saps their energy and makes them feel like—"

"Like crap!" Emily interrupted. "I know exactly what that feels like!"

"That's why planning is a must!"

"Hey, if water can accomplish everything you say it can and make me feel so much better, I'll happily become crazy enough to schedule it!" Emily exclaimed, as she circled her ear with her index finger and raised her other hand.

"Now when do we schedule the wine—I mean, water?" Emily joked. "Should I spread out my consumption over the entire day?"

"Yes, exactly. That's why it requires some forethought. Everyone has a different flow to their day. There's not a one-size that fits all. Some people like to sip water all day long. I like to guzzle about 12-14 ounces about every 3 hours.

"And remember to take your water bottle with you when you exercise. You'll want to drink before, during, and after exercise to compensate for the water you lose through respiration and sweat."

Emily looked hopeful, "Okay, that seems very doable. Start my day with water which will give me some momentum for good decisions throughout the rest of the day. Establish a cup that works for me, BPA-free, probably stainless steel, and a manageable size that I can refill several times. And lastly, make a plan for when I will drink it, preferably around every 3 hours! Consider it done!" Emily paused as she contemplated these new habits. "But how do I make sure I *remember* to drink at my planned times? I mean, my days are very full and I've been known to look for my reading glasses when they're sitting on top of my head!"

"I've done that a time or two myself. Here's the answer." I held up my phone. "Set the alarm on your phone."

"Seriously? An alarm?"

"I promise it will help you! After all these years, I still use daily reminders. I like the 6 A.M., 9 A.M., 12 P.M., 3 P.M., and 6 P.M. schedule for my water and I use quiet alarms to help me remember. Whether phone alarms, Fitbit tracking, computer reminders or even apps like Cozi that manage important appointments, most of us need a little help to remember important details through the day. Our schedules are just too busy to focus on water breaks. Why not make it easy on yourself? I really think you would like it once you got used to it. Want to give it a whirl?"

"Yeah, I guess it's worth a try...my family is going to think I've lost my marbles," Emily said, shaking her head.

"But you'll feel tons better, have a greater chance at losing weight, and literally affect every part of your day. Isn't that worth shaking things up a bit?"

"Absolutely—shake away! I'm so ready to feel better."

"Great, Emily! Now, here's your homework before we meet again next week. I want you to start using your planner tonight. Read the entire Introduction and start with Day 1. Then I want you to start implementing everything we talked about today.

"I promise, Emily. Over time this small habit will produce big results and that can help change your life."

Emily gently nodded, "I'm counting on it...more than you know."

Chapter 3
Sleep Like a Baby

One week later, I met up with Emily for our second training session. I greeted her cheerfully as we walked toward each other in the hallway. "Good morning, Emily! How are you feeling since we last saw each other?"

With hope written all over her face, Emily was bursting at the seams to update me on her success. What an awesome way to start my day!

"You'll be happy to know I consistently used my new tool every day last week! Can you believe it? And the 3 strategies you taught me made all the difference in tracking my water without forgetting about it. I set it up on my phone as an appointment and that worked like a charm. And even though it's only been a week, I seem to have more zip in the afternoon which is usually my lowest energy of the day. I don't feel perfect yet, but it's definitely better. I'm peeing *a lot*—and I'm not even mad about it!" Emily said, chuckling.

"I'm so glad you're not mad!" I responded, laughing.

"But more importantly, I'm so thrilled you noticed significant improvements in your energy and how you feel throughout the day. That will give you some phenomenal momentum as you tackle the second tool toward achieving crazy-good, feel-like-a-million-bucks energy.

"Well I'm all for that! Let's go! What is it?"

"Okay! You're sure you're ready?"

"Yeeeeees! Come on already!" Emily prodded.

"It's sleep!!"

The silence was deafening. Crickets again. Talk about a party buster.

"I know it's not rocket science, right? But trust me. Many, many people struggle with this to the point where it's a terrible battle every night and they feel overwhelming exhaustion all day long. It's extremely discouraging for them. And I know this is a problem for you too since you noted on your Healthy Checklist that you get less than 7 hours of sleep a night. Everyone needs a restful night of sleep to feel and live their best so that's what we're going to tackle next."

"I guess I thought sleep issues were just par for the course from stress, intense work pressures, and being middle-aged. I never thought there was much I could do about it. I certainly never thought this would be one of the 4 tools I needed to "change my life," but I am so incredibly tired of tossing and turning at night and ready to try anything that will help," Emily admitted. "Honestly I feel like I'm awake over half the night and that cannot be helping anything!"

"Absolutely it doesn't! Matter of fact, it can wreak havoc on your entire day and your long term health! But just like the strategies to increase your water were simple and practical, the way we approach sleep will be exactly the same. Simple. Doable. Easy to commit to so you should notice improvements fairly quickly. It's nearly impossible to be our best at work or pleasant to others all day long when we lay awake and stare at the ceiling all night, then feel frustrated and wrung out all day long."

"Yep, that's me, Laurie. I spend a good part of the day being ticked about not sleeping."

"Lots of folks share this problem with you, Emily. It seems we are getting a lot less sleep than we did just two generations ago. A 2013 survey from the *Gallup Poll* found that 41% of Americans don't get enough sleep to be healthy. Only 59% of U.S. adults did meet the standard of 7 to 9 hours, but in 1942, 84% did![1]

You've probably heard the word *hangry*, when you're so hungry you're angry about it. There's a new word in town to describe its cousin, being so tired and exhausted it makes you angry. Have you ever heard the word *slangry*?"

Emily looked at me with her head cocked as if I were making up a new word.

"I'm not kidding—it's already in the urban dictionary! Lack of sleep is becoming a serious problem that can have detrimental effects over your emotions, your relationships, your productivity during the day, your ability to remember details, and even your self-discipline when it comes to how much you eat. People who are sleep-deprived struggle with one or all of these symptoms—and now we have the word *slangry* to describe it. The fact is, going without enough sleep colors every part of your life and can really make you feel and act awful.

"And you can feel terribly angry and defeated when your brain won't shut off at a time when it should be sleeping. Then to make matters even worse, your whirling thoughts can punish you for hours with a long list of to-dos that you didn't accomplish. Or worry can keep you anxious replaying all the *what-ifs* involving your kids, job, marriage, health, aging parents, retirement—there's a long list. Not only can your thoughts keep you awake, night sounds like sirens, loud cars, house noises, a snoring spouse, or even the neighbor's barking dog can affect your quality of snoozing and keep you from falling asleep.

"Then there's the other group of folks who effortlessly drift into *la-la land* only to be awoken halfway through the night for a myriad of reasons with every attempt to fall back asleep completely derailed. They can fall asleep. They just can't *stay* asleep. Too often they spend the rest of the night full of anxiety or punching their pillow with frustration.

"Or, Emily, perhaps you've been tempted, as I have been, to hope that you could get by with a lot less sleep! Think of all the extra work you could get done!"

"It sure would simplify my work day!"

"Apparently lots of people have thought that very same thing because there are blogs, YouTube videos, and even t-shirts on the Internet that are selling the logo *Sleep Is for Suckers!*"

"Wow, I've never heard of that! But I have wished from time to time that I could get by on a lot less."

"I totally understand, Emily. We all want to accomplish more in each day. But if we try to function with only a few hours of sleep it can produce terrible consequences. Sleep-deprivation is not a badge of honor. It violates the way God created us, which is to get deep and restful sleep every night, for the right length of time. If God rested on the seventh day of creation in a great attempt to show us that we should do the same, why do we do everything in our power to avoid it?"

"Yeah, that's a good point," Emily agreed. "I still like the idea of getting more work done instead of sleeping," she said winking.

"Emily, I think we can find a way to do both! Productivity and rest can co-exist and even help each other. But unfortunately we live in an age of overwork and under-rest and it is taking a toll. I've even heard of companies that keep cots available for managers who work late into the night so they can catch a couple of winks before they do it all over again at the crack of dawn. That is crazy! We can't live like that! At least for very long—or very well. One of the most surprising trends I've noticed in recent years is that so few people sleep more than 7 hours!

"This is a widespread problem that is greatly affecting our health. Sleepless nights produce tons of anxiety. And anxiety disrupts quality and length of sleep. Disrupted sleep causes the pattern to start all over again. Guaranteed. It's a terrible and exhausting cycle to be on. Sleep is a great gift and a tool that is crucial to having extraordinary energy and health. That's why we're going to discuss it in detail."

"I've always been curious about all this stuff. Anything that can make me feel better is something I need to know a lot more about!"

"Great, Emily! Let's jump in.

"Sleep is critical and essential for your overall health since there's a lot of fundamental and key work going on while you're catching some zzz's. That's why inadequate sleep dramatically affects our quality of work. I wonder, of the 41% of people who struggle to sleep enough, how many fall asleep at work like I used to?!"

"Guilty!" Emily confessed as she raised her hand. "I'm glad it's not just me."

"Apparently insomnia is costing the U.S. an astounding $63.2 billion a year in lost productivity. Ronald Kessler, renowned professor and psychiatric epidemiologist at Harvard Medical School states, "Sleep deprivation is an underappreciated problem. Americans are not missing work because of insomnia. They are still going to their jobs but accomplishing less because they're woefully tired. In an information-based economy, it's difficult to find a condition that has a greater effect on productivity."[2k]

"Sleep-deprivation noticeably affects work productivity through *decreased* ability to think clearly, react quickly, form memories, feel alert, as well as concentrate and focus."

"Okay, so I'm a little foggy in the afternoon. Isn't everybody?" Emily asked.

"You don't have to be. What if you could get enough sleep to make your afternoons as productive as your mornings? What if you had enough energy and concentration to finish your projects *before* your deadlines? Wouldn't that feel amazing?"

Emily raised one eyebrow. I had piqued her interest. "Yeah, it would feel amazing. Do you have some extra focus and concentration in your back pocket?"

"No, but I bet *you* will very soon."

"Eternal optimist," Emily whispered under her breath.

"Yes, I am. I have great faith in you, your determination, and your courage to change. I know you don't want to suffer from *any* side effects of sleep deprivation which also include irritability, mood swings, relational conflict, anxiety, depression, illness, high blood pressure, heart disease, diabetes and accidents."

"Wow, I thought sleep deprivation just made me cranky."

"There's more. Losing sleep can also increase your chances of getting sick. According to Dr. Eric J. Olson, doctor of internal medicine in Rochester, Minnesota, "Lack of sleep can affect your immune system. Studies show that people who don't get quality sleep or *enough* sleep are more likely to get sick after being exposed to a virus, such as the common cold. Lack of sleep can also affect how fast you recover if you do get sick. During sleep, your immune system releases proteins called cytokines. Certain cytokines need to increase when you have an infection or inflammation. Sleep deprivation may *decrease* production of these protective cytokines. In addition, infection-fighting antibodies and cells are reduced during periods when you don't get enough sleep. So, your body needs enough sleep to effectively fight infectious diseases.[3]

"And if that weren't enough, lack of sleep is also now being associated with weight gain."

"What???? Whoa, whoa, whoa. Back up. Did you say *weight gain?*" Emily asked in disbelief.

"I know, the two don't seem connected at all, but surprisingly they are! A brain that is tired appears to crave high-carb, sugary snacks while decreasing the ability to say no to the impulse."

"No way! This is terrible news!"

"Yes, way, Emily. Many studies have produced those exact results! It was found that participants short on sleep had reduced leptin and elevated ghrelin. The hunger hormone ghrelin increases your appetite for high-calorie foods that stimulate the brain's reward centers. It also decreases your sensitivity to leptin, a hormone that shuts off hunger. A sleepy brain has a decreased ability to detect satiety and shut the appetite switch off. You can find this in several studies like the *American Planner of Clinical Nutrition.*"

"Oh that is just awesome news."

"I know, right? Sleep-deprivation can be a huge problem, not just to us, but to others as well," I explained to Emily. "Sleep-deprived people who were tested using a driving simulator or performing hand-eye coordination tasks did as badly as, or worse than, people who were intoxicated. In 2011, the *National Highway Traffic Safety Administration* released an article that stated in 2009, 72,000 crashes were a result of drowsiness."[4]

"Wow, that is alarming."

"One of the most catastrophic accidents in our U.S. history was the Challenger explosion in 1986. President Ronald Reagan appointed *The*

Rogers Commission to do an investigation on the cause. Their findings, to the best of their knowledge at the time, attributed the error to the severe sleep deprivations of the *NASA* managers."[5]

"Oh, my word! I had no idea. Sleep-deprivation is real and no one is immune." Emily paused, shaking her head. "I don't know why I think it doesn't affect me. It obviously influences my mood, my energy, health, relationships, concentration—my weight. Maybe this is a bigger deal than I've allowed myself to believe."

"Emily, the problem is that we get so used to being tired it's easy to forget the serious trouble it can bring. I think it warrants a closer look at why we actually need sleep and what happens to us when we rest."

"That's a plan. Talk fast, would you, so we can get to the good stuff. I want to know what I can change so I can actually sleep in my bed instead of toss all night."

I was happy to hear Emily's enthusiasm, even if it meant speed talking. "I'll do my best," I assured her.

"Emily, your body has a natural clock called a *circadian clock* which helps regulate your sleep. The word *circadian* refers to rhythmic biological cycles. They've also been called *circadian rhythms*—and they repeat at approximately 24-hour intervals."

"Yes, I've heard of those. Are they the same for everyone?"

"Everyone has *circadian rhythms* that are controlled by the hypothalamus region of the brain," I answered, "but each person's clock is set to their own schedule specifically.

"Light makes your hypothalamus sends out signals to different regions of the brain such as the pineal gland. The pineal gland shuts down the production of melatonin, which is a hormone that causes you to be drowsy and sleepy. That's why you're awake during the day.

"Your levels of melatonin naturally increase in the evening from lack of light and that's why you start to feel increasingly more tired as it gets darker in the evening."

"Ok, I'm with you. That explains why I felt more energetic on vacation last month in Hawaii. We had constant sunlight and I'm used to being in an office all day without a window."

"Well, yeah—that, and the fact that it was *Hawaii*. That couldn't have hurt your energy levels either."

"Nope, it didn't hurt one bit," Emily replied, grinning from ear to ear.

"The right *amount* of light is also important. I have a friend who lives in northern Alaska and she finds it very difficult to sleep in the summer months when they have 80 days of uninterrupted daylight. The opposite is true in winter when they have 67 days of sustained darkness with no sunlight at all."

Emily looked off into the distance. "I've always wanted to go to Alaska. It's so beautiful."

"Focus, focus," I reminded her. "We're almost to the *good part*."

Emily laughed and nodded her head, "I'm listening, coach!"

"Let's start by looking at the different levels of sleep. First, there are two main types of sleep: Non-Rapid Eye Movement (NREM) Sleep, which is also called quiet sleep, and Rapid Eye Movement (REM) Sleep, which is called active sleep."

"That's right. REM is when people dream and if you pull up one of their eyelids their eyes are darting like crazy!" Emily giggled, obviously speaking from experience. My raised eyebrows begged an explanation.

"I had younger siblings. It's part of the deal!" Emily confessed, smiling.

"REM sleep is only one phase of sleep. Your brain actually cycles through four phases of varying degrees of sleep."

"Hmmm, I thought I had heard there were five stages."

"Some sleep experts recently combined stages three and four, which are both deep sleep, but every phase is necessary to ensure that both your body and mind rest, recover, and rebuild themselves each night."

"I bet stage one has those big twitches," Emily said snickering. "Those are hilarious. My husband is notorious for those when he's napping in his chair. Ranger, our dog, will crawl up on his lap and fall asleep so the two of them are all cozy and quiet—until Jeffrey has a gigantic twitch and they both practically jump through the ceiling! Now that's some funny stuff right there."

"That's right, Emily. It can produce some comical moments if you're the one awake and watching it. Your body begins with Non-REM sleep, which is about 75% of all your sleep. In stage one, your brain is beginning to slow down and relax. You're not really in a deep sleep yet but you are out of it enough to experience possible myoclonic jerks which is where you are suddenly startled. My husband is famous for these as well and usually thinks he is slipping on ice. Twitching is very common during this stage and lasts a very brief time, generally 5 to 10 minutes. This is also the stage where you think you can change the television channel on someone who looks asleep, and then they speak up and say, 'Hey, I was watching that.'"

Emily laughed, "Oh my, yes. Jeffrey says that exact thing every time I try to change his baseball game to *HGTV*."

"Well, maybe you should wait until you can pull up his eyelids," I teased.

"Good point. Duly noted." Emily nodded.

"The next level is stage two and lasts for approximately 20 to 30 minutes. Your body temperature starts to decrease, your heart rate begins to slow, and you become disengaged from your surroundings. At this stage you are lightly sleeping," I explained.

I could see Emily's wheels turning. "Should I change the television channel yet?" she asked.

"Probably not yet, but definitely in the next two stages," I replied.

"Okay, good. It doesn't take very long to get to stage three...about 30 to 40 minutes?" Emily asked.

"Yes," I said, "but remember everyone is a little bit different and each sleep episode is slightly unique so keep that in mind before you poke a sleeping bear."

Emily lit up. "I know, I'll set the timer," she said, amusing herself. "I've got this timer thing down since I've been using it for my water. Now I use it for everything."

I wasn't quite sure what she meant by *everything* but I was very pleased to hear she was loving the idea of using her alarm.

"Stage three is when you become less responsive to noises. This stage plays a major role in your health and is eventually where the deepest and most restorative sleep occurs. This is your VIP sleep. You're probably not getting enough of this stage, Emily, which is why you wake up so tired. During this stage your blood pressure drops, breathing rate slows, muscles relax, tissue is repaired, muscles and bones are built, your immune system is strengthened, and energy is restored. You're likely to feel disoriented if you wake unexpectedly while you're in this phase.

"Now here's an interesting fact—at the end of this stage is where sleepwalking and bed-wetting and are most likely to occur."

Emily snickered and said, "Yeah, I don't really have a problem with that anymore. As you know, I've been peeing a ton more with all my water-drinking—just not in the bed."

"Even though obviously you don't have to worry about bed-wetting, a lot of kids do struggle with bed-wetting so this could be helpful information for your colleagues or co-workers who have young kids. It does affect your life if you're surrounded by people who are not sleeping or who have anxiety because their kids are struggling with their sleep."

"Very true. Tell me more."

"We've learned a lot from studying the brain and researchers have discovered that kids don't wet the bed on purpose. The part of their brain that controls the urge to pee just hasn't developed yet. But there is a great remedy for it. I've seen dozens of families cure this problem in just a week or so by using a specific bed-wetting sensor and alarm. This teaches the brain to hold the pee so it doesn't have to wake up when it shouldn't, and the child stops peeing the bed for good. No medication. No shame. Just a simple alarm that changes the brain and helps it work better. And everybody gets more sleep. How great is that?"

"Yeah, it really is. Our brains are so amazing," Emily agreed.

"It's a remarkable invention," I said. "And while I know it's not a problem for you, now you can share the solution with your friends or co-workers that may have young children struggling with the issue. They'll thank you for helping them all sleep again."

"A rested worker is a productive worker, that's for sure! I've never heard of that alarm but it's genius. And now that you've solved the sleep problems of my co-workers, do you possibly have something in your magic bag for me?"

"Almost there. We just need to finish up with REM sleep. You know, the pull-up-the-eyelid stage."

Emily giggled, "I love that stage—it just conjures up so many fun memories!"

"And it's an important level of sleep as well. REM is where you dream, which makes up the remaining 25% of your sleep. This occurs approximately 70 to 90 minutes after you fall asleep and may only last about 10 minutes on the first cycle. Then you cycle back to a lighter stage and begin the process all the way to REM again about four to five times each night.

"This is where you have the greatest chance to successfully change the channel on Jeffrey. The brain is active and energized but the body is immobile and relaxed. The dream stage is extremely valuable to the quality of sleep you get. It's a sign that you are truly resting deeply."

"Okay, so this is the best time to change the channel, correct?"

"Or you could just ask him nicely while he's awake," I suggested.

Emily giggled. "Nah, its way more fun this way."

"So that's it for Sleep 101. Does this help explain why sleep-deprivation is a huge problem that can have dire consequences on your energy, mood, appetite, health, work, and relationships?

"I do better understand how my lack of sleep is totally screwing up my energy and everything else. Now the 60,000 dollar question—what are we going to do about it?"

"That's our next discussion, Emily. And there is a ton of "good stuff" to share. You ready to make some changes?

"Girl, I live ready," Emily replied confidently then quickly added, "right after a pee break."

Music to my ears.

Chapter 4
Sweet Dreams are Made of These

Jumping right in to the "good stuff", "Emily, I've noticed over the years that clients who struggled with sleep were sending the wrong signals to their brains *throughout the day*. Some of the common enemies of sleep can usually be found in what goes on during the day. That's really what holds the key to your struggles at night. You have to look at all the possible cues you send your brain that relay the wrong messages. Are you willing to dive that deep?"

"I am so willing—bring it on!"

"Great, Emily! The first step is to find out how much sleep you actually need. As you can see by this handy-dandy chart," I explained, as I pulled out the sleep level guide, "most adults need between 7-9 hours of sleep each night."

"Whoa, look at that!" Emily exclaimed as she looked over the chart. "That seems like a lot of sleep. There's no way I get that amount. Why is it so much?"

"That's how long it takes for your brain to run a few times through all the sleep cycles. This could be why your focus and ability to concentrate take a nosedive in the afternoons, especially now that you're drinking enough water. Once hydration is no longer a problem, you have to look at *how much* sleep you're getting.

"Do you wake feeling like you are ready to jump out of bed?"

"No. Hardly ever."

"Didn't you say you feel a bit foggy and sluggish in the afternoons?"

"Yes, sometimes," Emily said, as she contemplated her answer. "It's a little better with the water I'm drinking but it's still a struggle."

"Are you ever tired enough to nap?" I asked.

"Yes," Emily admitted. "There are so many days when I just want to put my head on my desk and close my eyes."

"Do you ever find yourself growing impatient or snapping at people because you're just dog-tired?"

Emily winked and said, "Well, yes. But it's hard to say *exactly* what causes that."

"You get where I'm going here. You need a lot more rest then you're currently getting. You, my friend, are sleep-deprived.

"According to the *National Institute of Neurological Disorders and Stroke*, adequate sleep needs are contingent on several factors, including age and stage of life.[1] In 2015, recommendations by researchers with the National Sleep Foundation released the following chart as a guide for sleep duration by age. These recommendations were based on a review of more than 300 research studies.

"The best way to discover how much sleep you actually need is to use a short period of time when you can go to bed at the same time every night and allow yourself to sleep until you wake up on your own, without an alarm. Obviously this would have to be during a time that you are on vacation from work or have a long weekend. If you have a sleep debt to begin with, it may take a few days before you're caught up. You will eventually discover how many hours of sleep are best for you and what time you would naturally wake up."

Age Group	Amount of Sleep Needed
Newborns (0 to 3 months)	14 to 17 hours per day
Infants (4 to 11 months)	12 to 15 hours
Toddlers (1 to 2 years)	11 to 14 hours
Preschoolers (3 to 5 years)	10 to 13 hours
School-age (6 to 13 years)	9 to 11 hours

Age Group	Amount of Sleep Needed
Teenagers (14 to 17 years)	8 to 10 hours
Adults (18 to 64 years)	7 to 9 hours
Pregnant Women	During pregnancy, women may need a few more hours of sleep per night or a few short naps during the day.
Older Adults (65 + years)	7 to 8 hours

"So, let me guess," Emily said. "You sleep a consistent 7 hours every night?"

"Nope, I sure don't."

"Aha! I knew it! See, no one sleeps that much!"

"I usually sleep 8 hours."

"Oh it just figures."

"It does give me an extra zip so I do try to give my body what it needs. Am I perfect? No. Do I *always* get 8 hours, pop out of bed like toast, and sing like a bird? Of course not. But I am very deliberate about achieving good quality rest on most nights because it affects *everything and every person* in my day. Every single meeting. Every single interaction. Every idea. Every phone call. I feel like a stronger, nicer, calmer, more productive person when I'm well-rested. And I know that's what you want, Emily, or you wouldn't be standing here with me. You want to be more energized, productive, and emotionally balanced through the day, right?"

"Yeah…"

"And feel extraordinary, right?"

"Yes," Emily said, smiling.

"And I want that for you too! So much of your sleep quality hinges on the cues you're sending to your brain so let's explore those messages and see what we can discover, shall we?"

"That's sounds like a plan, Sherlock," Emily teased.

Set the Stage during the Day

"First, how much movement do you get through the day? Exercise improves the quality of your sleep by using up surplus adrenaline that's released during daily stress, which all of us experience. Exercise helps you fall asleep faster, achieve deeper sleep, and awaken fewer times during the night because it reduces the amount of adrenaline circulating in your bloodstream. People who achieve daily moderate to vigorous exercise enjoy a 65% improvement in overall sleep quality."

"That's one of the big reasons I'm here," Emily admitted. "I know I need more exercise. I'm just not a big fan of it."

"You've got me in your corner, Emily. We all stay more motivated with the help of those around us and movement is extremely important to your quality of rest. Exercise is simply one of the greatest influencers over sleep there is. I often hear clients say they can predict the quality of their sleep at night by their exercise that day."

"I know I sleep better on the days I get out and walk. But frankly, after work I just don't have enough pep to feel like doing anything other than going home and putting up my feet."

"I completely understand that feeling. That's why we'll focus more on the mornings for you. There are quite a few benefits to scheduling exercise in the morning. It's another strong decision that boosts your willpower throughout the rest of the day. Plus, as you know, later in the day there are always more fires to put out both at work and home that can interfere with your ability to get to a gym or even take a walk."

"Yes, too many fires disrupt my best-laid plans," Emily freely confessed.

"As part of your homework, we're going to start you with a morning walking plan, 5 to 6 days a week, 20 minutes each time. And not just a stroll! You're going to put some power into it. Walk like you're really going somewhere—because you are, right? Sound good?"

"Not really..."

I shot a quick glance over to Emily to see if she was serious.

"Just kidding," Emily quickly piped back. "I'm all in, so yes, I promise to work hard—and walk like I'm going somewhere."

"Excellent, Emily. The second way to cue your brain during the day is to stop your intake of caffeine around noon. Caffeine is a stimulant that can interfere with your ability to fall asleep or sleep soundly. According to Roland Griffiths, PhD, a professor in the departments of psychiatry and neuroscience at the *Johns Hopkins University School of Medicine*, caffeine can also cause jitters, headaches, nervousness and irregular heartbeat. Coffee, tea, cola, cocoa, chocolate and some prescription and non-prescription drugs contain caffeine, and depending on the amount and the milligrams of the caffeine, can stay in your system for up to 14 hours![2] A 2007 *Consumer Reports* study found that even some decaf coffees contained caffeine, with one having 32 mg per cup—about the same amount as in 12 ounces of caffeinated soda!"[3]

Emily nodded her head and replied, "I know exactly what they mean! I've ordered decaf coffee in the afternoon thinking I would be fine and then couldn't fall asleep until 3 a.m.!"

"Exactly. And while the effects of caffeine are different for everyone, for some folks a single cup of coffee can mean a miserable, sleepless night—for others that might take 3 cups. Caffeine, being a diuretic, can also interrupt sleep by increasing the need to pee in the middle of the night.

"I know you love your coffee, Emily, and I do as well. But when it comes to getting better sleep, you have to be willing to shut off the flow at noon. Or you could try herbal tea in the afternoon which is naturally caffeine-free."

"Done," Emily replied without any deliberation.

Okay, THAT was easy. Let's hope the rest of it goes as well.

"The third way to get better sleep and correctly signal the brain during the day is to avoid nicotine. Stop smoking or chewing tobacco. Nicotine, like caffeine, is a central nervous system stimulant that can cause insomnia. Just like caffeine, nicotine can make it harder to fall asleep because it increases your heart rate, raises blood pressure, and stimulates brain activity. I know this all too well since my dad smoked every single day starting at the age of 16."

"I agree. It is completely unhealthy which is why I don't smoke."

"But didn't you say on your Healthy Checklist that your husband smokes in the car and occasionally chews tobacco?"

"Yes, but how does that affect *me*?"

"You're getting his second-hand smoke when you're with him which means you're ingesting a stimulant. And if he is also chewing tobacco and then can't fall asleep, he could be affecting your sleep by tossing and turning."

"Huh," Emily replied, thinking about their sleep habits. "Jeffrey does really struggle to fall asleep. It's frustrating for him and aggravating for me. I guess we've just been blaming it on our work stress but the truth is that he struggles even more than I do."

"I've had many clients kick the tobacco habit and they all notice they fall asleep more quickly and wake less often during the night."

"I'll have Jeffrey call you. That way we can both get some sleep!" Emily exclaimed. "Okay, what's next on the list?"

"The fourth way to prepare for sleep during the day is to make your days as bright as possible. Get some sunlight! This shuts down the production of the sleep inducing hormone melatonin. Since you spend long days at work where you're not exposed to natural sunlight, it can significantly impede your ability to stay awake."

"Light makes such a difference to me. I know I don't get enough during the day because I felt so different on vacation with all the sun I was getting."

"Hawaii. Yes, I know."

Emily laughed, "Hey, good memory. You must be getting enough sleep."

"The fifth way to cue the brain during the day is by getting up at the same time each morning. Your brain loves consistent, predictable routines and will respond by setting an automatic internal clock. After a while, your brain won't even need an alarm to wake up. Consistency is the key since a regular sleep schedule keeps the circadian rhythms synchronized.

"So what time do you get up in the morning, Emily?"

"Oh, it varies within about 30 minutes. Regardless of the time, I'm never ready to wake up. Isn't it more important what time I go to bed?"

"Actually, what time you need to get up determines what time you should go to bed," I explained. "Keep in mind that you are striving to reach at least the minimum of 7 hours of sleep."

"I need to be up by 7 and out the door by 8 o'clock."

"Starting tomorrow, Emily, we'll be pushing that back an hour since you'll be working out for 30 minutes every morning. So with a new wake time of 6 o'clock you'll need to fall asleep by at least 11 p.m."

"If you can get me to fall asleep by 11 p.m. you are a miracle worker. Wait, did you say I'll be working out every morning at 6 a.m.?"

"Yes, ma'am," I said as cheerfully as possible. "Working out at 6 AM is part of your new routine. If you diligently and consistently make the necessary lifestyle adjustments we've been discussing, I have no doubt we can get you to fall asleep by 11 p.m. each night. How would that feel?"

"That would feel amazing! I would do almost anything to finally get some sleep. Even get up at 6 AM! This will be challenging for sure—and I may be mad at you for a while—but I am doing this!"

"So those are some strategies to use *during the day*, helping you set the stage for good sleep at night."

"Okay, you're right. Those are all easy ways to signal my brain during the day—exercise, cut back on caffeine, and nicotine for Jeffrey, get up at the same time every day, and increase sunlight. Got it! Check, check, and check."

"Now that you've set the stage for good sleep during the day, you also have to send the right signals to your brain in your sleeping environment. Your bedroom sends out signals whether to sleep or be awake at night."

"You're saying my bedroom speaks to my brain?" Emily asked with exaggerated cynicism.

"Yep, it sends messages loud and clear," I responded confidently.

"Well then, do tell. I'm all ears so my bedroom can speak."
I think she was slightly mocking me, but attentive, nonetheless.

SET THE STAGE IN YOUR BEDROOM

"Your bedroom actually communicates to your brain in a very consistent and predictable pattern, for your good or for your detriment. You want to make sure it conveys a "sleep" message that registers with your brain and there are several factors that transmit this signal.

"First, we want to look at making sure your room is as *dark* as possible. The darker it is, the better you'll sleep. Cover electrical displays and anything that emits a light. Use heavy curtains or shades to block light from windows, or try a sleep mask to cover your eyes. If you wake up during the night to use the bathroom, keep the light to a minimum as long as it's safe to do so and you don't trip over anything. This will make it easier to go back to sleep.

"I've had many clients struggle with getting up in the middle of the night to use the bathroom and then couldn't get back to sleep because of the bright bathroom light. Once they started using a nightlight or a dimmer in the bathroom, they were able to immediately fall back asleep upon returning to bed. Darkness signals the brain to stay asleep. Bright lights cue your brain to wake up. It's just that simple."

Emily was listening intently and processing all the ideas I was suggesting. "So," she started, "I want to do the opposite of what I'm trying to do during the day?"

"Exactly, darkness is your friend." I replied. "The second tip is to make sure your bedroom is as *quiet* as possible. Some people sleep so soundly they wouldn't hear a train roll through their bedroom. While others can hear a leaf fall to the ground outside their window."

"That would be Jeffrey and me. He doesn't hear anything and I hear every blasted sound."

"The key for a person like you, Emily, with sensitive hearing, is to keep the sound consistent. It's often the random, loud noises that wake light-sleepers. It's almost impossible to eliminate all noise but many people have found relief by using ear plugs, a white noise machine, soothing noise apps, music on their phones, music from Alexa, or SMART house technology that offers the sound of waves. The key is to keep sound consistent."

"The third way your bedroom speaks to your brain is through the *temperature* in the room. It's important to keep your bedroom cool. A room that is either too warm or too cold can be uncomfortable to the point of disrupting sleep. Studies have shown that most people sleep best in a room that is around 65°F."

"A+ pupil right here!" Emily said proudly, pointing to herself. "We keep ours right at 65°F."

"Great, Emily! That will help you so much."

"The fourth way to cue your brain to sleep requires you to examine the obvious—your bed. Make sure your bed is perfectly comfortable and that includes your mattress, pillow, and bedding. Think of yourself as *Goldilocks*—your bed should be just right for *you*.

"I've been telling Jeffrey for quite some time that we need a new mattress! We usually end up sinking toward each other in the middle. Then we flop around like fish out of water trying to get comfortable and it takes a ridiculous amount of time to settle in."

"Oh my word, that sounds frustrating. Why don't you just invest in a new mattress?"

"And that is the big $60,000 question! We know we need it. We just haven't made time for it. It's terrible trying to fall asleep on a soft, unsupportive, and sinking mattress. A new mattress obviously needs to go on my to-do list *today*!"

"Memory foam toppers can work well too if a mattress is too firm, but it sounds like yours has lived its life and it's time to replace it. Also check your pillows. Use only a pillow that perfectly supports your neck. It should be so comfortable that you don't even notice it. I prefer very firm memory foam but everyone is different."

"I'm starting to feel like the *Princess and the Pea*," Emily mused.

"That's really okay. The point is to be as comfortable as possible because it does greatly affect your sleep. If you're going to spend one third of your life in bed trying to get a good night's sleep that affects your entire day, it may as well be in a bed that is perfect for you!"

"Very good point. We'll do some shopping as soon as possible."

"The fifth way to correctly cue your brain in your bedroom is to stay in bed if you wake up during the night. Remember that you cycle from light to heavy sleep, back and forth, and sometimes you may wake during the light sleep cycle. That doesn't mean you should get out of bed. If you're waking up during the night and having trouble falling back asleep, by all means, don't turn to your iPad or phone or work. Do your best to relax and stay in bed which cues your brain to sleep."

"The sixth tip is to train your brain to recognize what it means when you go to bed. Teach your brain to know that going to bed means either *sex or sleep*. Avoid using your bed to catch up on work. Insomnia can often be the result of stress and anxiety so make sure bedtime cues your brain to relax."

"So, you're saying I can train my brain to know *why* I'm in bed?"

"Have you ever heard of Pavlov's dog?" I asked Emily.

"Yes, of course. That's the story about the dog, the bell, and the food, right?"

"Yes, the bell meant food was being served. After a while, the dog's brain was so well trained to expect food when he heard the bell that he would salivate every time he heard the bell even when food was not given."

"How does that relate to training my brain for bed? Do I need a bell?" Emily asked, jokingly.

"The bell is symbolic. The purpose of that story is to remind us how quickly the brain adapts to recurring experiences and how it will anticipate the same results from constant stimuli.

"I'll do my best to retrain my brain to anticipate sleep or sex, not work, when I get into bed. It will definitely be a stretch but if I'm going to do all these other things in an effort to sleep better, I'm sure not going to be weak here!"

"Excellent, Emily. That's the spirit! Easy-peasy. Now let's look at the signals you send your brain at the *end of the day.*"

"I think a glass of wine at the end of the day sends the perfect signal," Emily winked.

"Let's see if it works," I responded, winking back.

SET THE STAGE IN THE EVENING

"Your evenings are a very important time to tell your brain to sleep. We can accomplish this in two different ways: eliminate and prepare. We want to *eliminate* the enemies of sleep that can be found in what we drink, eat, and view. Then we want to *prepare* our minds, bodies, and hearts to enter into a deeply relaxed state to we can effortlessly drift into sweet dreams and sleep soundly the entire night. How's that sound, Emily?"

"Like a dream."

"I thought it might. So let's start with what is helpful to *eliminate* at night, specifically in what you drink.

"Did you know alcohol can actually keep you awake in the middle of the night?"

"What??? What's wrong with a little wine at dinner?"

"If you go to bed at 11 p.m., then your last drink should be no later than 8 p.m. Let me explain why. Most people think alcohol will help them sleep better. But it actually can greatly *interrupt* sleep. The sugar content in wine can wake you in the middle of the night when you should be sleeping deeply and dreaming. It can actually make insomnia worse."

"Worse?" Emily asked, shaking her head. "Well I don't need that. I can have a glass earlier in the night, right?"

"Yes," I replied. "One glass should not disturb your deep sleep, as long as it's early enough."

"Okay, cut back on the wine late at night. What else?"

"It also matters what you *eat* before bedtime as well. Limit large and spicy meals at dinner. They can leave your digestive system working overtime and actually interfere with your sleep. Try to make dinnertime earlier in the evening and avoid heavy, rich foods within 2 hours of bed. Fatty foods and large meals require a lot of work for your stomach to digest and often make sleep difficult."

"Guilty as charged," Emily confessed. "We eat our biggest meal at the end of the day and we often have indigestion as we lie in bed. Okay, eliminate large meals and spicy foods."

"Also what you *view* in the form of electronics has an impact on your sleep since they emit blue lights that stimulate your brain and decrease melatonin."

"And I need melatonin to fall asleep and sleep deeply, right?"

"You got it, Em. Try to eliminate all electronics about an hour before bed.

"And, you know," I added, "we found in our family our electronics were keeping us from not only good sleep but also from ending our day in meaningful conversation, praying together, sharing what we're thankful for, and focusing on all the good."

"That does sounds like a much better way to end an evening than working on my iPad until my eyes are burning from exhaustion. I'm going to try that thankful part. It's got to be better than my current plan."

"I know it will help tremendously, Emily. Plus, it's part of your homework so now you really have to do it."

"I'm ready, willing, and able to tackle all the things that need to be eliminated. But what should I do for the "prepare" part of better sleep?"

"The 'preparation' part are the things you *add* that help you sleep. You can do this by **developing some bedtime rituals** that promote relaxation and signal the end of the day. Sleep experts call this final phase "Bedtime Hygiene" meaning a set of practices that help you sleep better.

"We do this for our kids with bath time, reading stories, saying bedtime prayers, kissing everyone goodnight—why do we stop doing a version of this as adults? Developing bedtime rituals sends a very strong message to the brain that it's time to relax and fall asleep. Gary

Zammit, PhD, director of *Sleep Disorders Institute* in New York says that 'Bedtime rituals significantly help your brain shift into sleep mode.'[6]

"Everyone likes something different so try a few of these to see what works best for you.

"**Try soaking in a hot bath** for 20 minutes. Joyce Walsleben, PhD, Associate Professor at *New York University School of Medicine* says that if you raise your temperature a degree or two with a bath, the steeper drop at bedtime is likely to put you in a deep sleep. A shower is less effective apparently, but can work in a pinch."[4]

"You could also try adding Epsom Salt to your bath time. According to the *Epsom Salt Council*, the magnesium in Epsom salt may aid in improved sleep by helping muscles and nerves relax and also reducing inflammation to relieve pain and muscle cramps. And the sulfates in Epsom salts can help flush toxins, which always makes it easier to relax."[5]

"I never take baths. They just seem like a lot of work and waste of time."

"There are lots of bedtime rituals to choose from. This is just one that has worked well for others and has some research to back it up so it might be worth a try.

"I guess it couldn't hurt," Emily replied, shrugging her shoulders.

"That's the spirit," I said, trying to acknowledge every step forward.

"Drinking herbal tea, particularly chamomile, can be relaxing. You can also try rubbing on some coconut oil and Shea butter for moisturizer, listening to soft music, reading a devotional, practicing stretching and relaxation techniques, using essential oils—all those can be useful in relieving tension and setting the stage to sleep."

"I love all those things and I'm sure they would serve me better than working all night. A little Andrea Bocelli, some herbal tea, relaxation techniques, and essential oils? That does sound very appealing. Do you have any suggestions for how to best use the oils?"

"According to Certified Aromatherapist Kayla Fioravanti, essential oils should be diluted in carrier oil, lotion, soap, bath salts or other modes of application. Lavender or clary sage, in particular, seem to help promote relaxation.[7]

"Regardless of what you add to your routine, the most important component of establishing a bedtime ritual is just starting somewhere! You can add whatever rituals you like."

"Wow! If I'm supposed to be asleep by 11 PM, I probably need to start all these bedtime rituals at 9!"

"Emily," I said calmly. "This is not a work project or competition. There's no extra credit for getting them all done. The idea is to pick and choose some of the habits that you find most soothing. Make up your own routine but try to give it a calm and peaceful flow. You're trying to de-stress here, not get more worked up. Let it be peace-filled. Take a deep breath and let it be for you. Your spirit. Your body. Your relaxation."

"You're right. It's not a project or a competition. I guess it's just hard for me to calm my brain down. No wonder I can't sleep at night."

"Emily, you have permission to treat yourself with kindness. It's not a luxury—it truly is a necessity. You're teaching your brain to destress so you can have much better sleep each night. That's the only way to be your best for everyone else.

"Okay, that leaves us one last bedtime ritual. Are you still with me?"

Emily nodded and said "Lay it on me, sister."

Did she just call me sister? How far we had come in such a short time! I wanted to jump up and click my heels.

"Before we go over this last one, I want to first assign your homework. Tonight I want you to begin establishing your bedtime rituals—and remember it's not a project. Secondly, I want you to make a list each night of all the things for which you are thankful. Thirdly, I want you to start shopping for a new mattress."

Emily laughed, "Got it! I might just try *all* of the bedtime rituals tonight!" Emily noticed I had one eyebrow raised and added, "I know, I know. Not a competition."

"Okay, the final way to prepare for sleep is to **manage your thoughts**. So often anxious thoughts are rooted in fear. Fear leads to worry, worry to stress, and stress leads to sleepless nights. If you find yourself lying awake worrying about things beyond your control or convinced that the worst-case-scenario in situations will come true, you can make yourself utterly miserable."

Emily agreed. "I'm pretty much a worry wart about my kids and work. There just always seems to be an issue I'm dealing with or some serious problem I have to solve. How do I quiet my spirit in the midst of all that? This pace is killing me. My heart seems to race uncontrollably at night when it should be helping me relax, right? And as much as I grouse about slowing down, I spend a lot of time solving other people's problems and it makes my head spin to the point I feel nauseated. By the time I do calm down enough to sleep, it's flippin' time to get up! I know I need to work on *all* the areas you've talked about, but this last one," Emily paused as she took a deep breath, "it resonates in every part of me. I really need help finding some peace, ya know?"

Emily's deep look of concern told me this was hitting a nerve well beyond needing "sleep tips." This was a matter of finding deep and healing respite for her soul. "For me," I said, trying to be as honest as possible, "I find that there is great peace when I finally admit, 'I can't carry this burden or fix that problem. I can't change situations that are painful or take away the suffering of those I love.' When I'm finally willing to admit that the burdens I'm carrying are too much for me, I start to feel a lift. A hope. A reassurance that I don't have to fix things. What can I do? I can pray. I can ask God to help me. And he tells me what to think about instead."

"And what's that? What are we supposed to be thinking about?" Emily asked anxiously.

"Well, it's not fear apparently. There are 365 references in the Bible where God says, 'Do not fear.'"

"Wow, one for each day. Like that was a coincidence."

"It was God's way of saying no matter what you face *every single day*, I've got you and you don't have to be afraid. You're not alone.

"He also says in Philippians 4:6, 'Don't worry about *anything*; instead pray about everything. Tell me what you need, and thank me for all I've done.' So that becomes my purpose instead of worrying. I focus on telling God what I need him to handle—and sometimes the list is very long. Sometimes it's so painful I can't speak it out loud. Sometimes I whisper it between my tears."

"Really?" Emily asked, surprised. "You seem so happy—all the time. Like nothing bothers you. Ever."

"You know, Emily, there just isn't a person alive that goes through this life without disappointment, discouragement, and heartbreak. I've learned if I rely on myself to handle it, I worry myself sick. Literally. It makes me physically sick. Thirty years ago that's all I knew how to do. Worry. But now I've learned that when I pour it all out to God—all the yuck this world throws at us, all the emotional gut punches, just all it— I'm flooded with peace. A divine and holy peace that can only come from His love. Then I make a list of all my blessings and I thank Him for every single thing I can think of. And that's what fills up the hurting places in my mind and heart instead of fear."

Emily was taking in all in. Then almost in a whisper, she asked, "And then what?"

"That's it. I pray. I know I'm loved. I thank Him for all the good in my life and I fall asleep with that covering me."

"Well," Emily whispered quietly, "what if you don't feel like praying—or know how? I mean, what do I even say?"

"Emily, you can talk to God any time, any place. Seriously. I pray here in the gym all the time. He loves his kids like we love ours—only a gazillion times more! He loves your voice. He loves your heart. He loves everything about you. Ask Him to help you. To fill you with peace—and He will!"

"Can I do that right now? Don't we need to be in a church or something?"

"I think this is church, Emily.

"Besides, you didn't pick me as your trainer by coincidence. He wanted you to know that the best way to have extraordinary sleep and rest is to have His extraordinary peace."

Emily had tears in her eyes as she touched my shoulder. "I knew it wasn't a coincidence."

So we prayed together in the training room of that gym surrounded by barbells, treadmills, disco music—and Jesus.

Oh, sweet Jesus, you are tender to the cries of those seeking you. No matter where they are. No matter where they've been. You are near and you answer with love.

As we opened the door to leave, Emily hugged me tightly and whispered, "You were so right, Laurie. This is going to change my life forever."

You can count on it. Sister.

Chapter 5
Get Movin'!

I couldn't wait to see Emily again. It had been a week since our last meeting that had ended in prayer and I just knew things were going to be very different for her. Laying down the heaviness of worry and daily choosing peace changes us in a profound way. I knew it would Emily start flexing her confidence muscle. Unshakeable commitment would be her new voice. Consistency, her dear friend. Not the kind of friend that says, "Let's skip our workout and drink wine." Nope, the kind of friend that says "We're doing this together—let's get our sweat on—cus' it will be so worth it!" A breakthrough was giving her courage to try new things. Just in time too. She was going to need divine strength to embrace our next discussion.

At week three, we were halfway through the 4-week program. But I also knew we were starting even greater challenges for Emily as we tackled the subjects of exercise and food. With water and sleep already under Emily's belt, I felt confident we could approach week three with the same grit and determination. A little coaxing might be in order, so I decided to include one of her favorite places in our discussion as we came to grips with perhaps her toughest battle so far.

So why not start with, in my opinion, one of the most beautiful places on earth? Hawaii. It is drop-dead gorgeous! The dramatic waterfalls, picturesque beaches, and stunning tropical gardens are truly extraordinary. Mike and I had an opportunity to visit on our 10-year anniversary and since then I refer to Hawaii as my adult Disney World. It's magical from the moment you arrive and have a lei placed around your neck at the airport until the moment you bid adieu to the fragrant and exotic paradise in the middle of the Pacific Ocean. It seems no one ever wants to leave. And many don't.

Mike and I were amazed to meet so many folks that visited for their vacation and never left. Some of them gave up very lucrative careers to open a t-shirt shop on the north end of Oahu. Others sold their companies on the mainland, trading the board room for selling surfboards. A lot of their decisions didn't make sense to me until I spent a little time inhaling the Hawaiian *Hakuna-Matata,* no-worries lifestyle. It focused on one thing—enjoying the exquisite beauty of paradise as it invaded one's soul with glorious inspiration and tranquility.

Yes. Hawaii was just the ticket to jumpstart Emily's third week.

We were at a tipping point. I knew Emily would never experience optimal results in her health without finding a form of movement that she liked enough to keep doing. She had already made it clear that exercise was not high on her priority list. Translation: she would avoid it every chance she got unless I could convince her otherwise. I admit, exercise can be a tough sell sometimes. What's to love about getting all sweaty, stinky, and exhausted? It prepares you to conquer mountains! That's what.

"Emily, hey, good morning!" I said cheerfully, greeting her at 6 AM on the nose.

She smiled and surprisingly greeted me with equal enthusiasm. "Hi there! What's on the docket this beautiful morning?"

We were off to a good start.

"I know how much you love Hawaii," I started, "so I thought I would share a story from one of my trips there."

"Wonderful. I'd love to hear it," she replied, as she sat down and gave me her full attention.

"I absolutely love hiking with my husband. And what better place than Hawaii, right?"

"Absolutely. There's hiking for days—if you're into that kind of thing," Emily said, laughing.

"Which we are," I said, smiling and nodding my head. "And the mother of them all is Diamond Head. It has a trail that will take you all the way to the top!"

"Wow, the closest I ever got to Diamond Head was seeing it from the veranda of the Pink Palace as I sipped a Mai Tai," she said chuckling. "So how was it?"

"It was a strenuous climb, to say the least. But the anticipation of the panoramic beauty of the Pacific Ocean with its crystal clear, blue water stretching for as far as the eye could see truly made it exhilarating! Really beyond description. I couldn't wait to get to the top, even with sweat dripping off every part of me."

"You were dripping sweat? And you liked it? There's something a little strange about you, lady."

Emily loved to poke fun at my passion for all things healthy but I knew I was getting through to her. I continued painting the picture of one of our favorite places on earth. "After an hour of hiking, sometimes straight uphill, Mike and I finally arrived at the top of the crater, exhausted and elated all at the same time! We were completely overwhelmed by the exquisite, breathtaking views. Even Pearl Harbor, several miles away, was clearly visible along the palm tree coastline nestling Waikiki Beach. The magnificence was truly mesmerizing. There wasn't much to say—we were in total awe."

"That's fantastic! I bet it was over-the-top gorgeous!" Emily exclaimed.

Little did she know, I was preparing her for a spectacular bucket-list challenge of her own.

"It was incredible, Emily. But what made it *most* memorable is the person we met on the way up."

"Oh, wow, did you meet Oprah?" she asked, excitedly. "She has a house there, you know. Or maybe Clint Eastwood? I think he lives there too. Did you get a picture?"

"No, it wasn't Oprah or Clint—or anyone famous. Although I will never forget her."

"So who was she?"

"Before I reveal that, let me first start by explaining the design of the trail. When we started at the bottom, the pathway initially offered a 10-foot wide concrete sidewalk, beckoning even the most novice hiker with a smooth and easy route. It made us think *this is going to be a walk in the park*. But then, about 35 minutes into the ascent, the trail suddenly squeezed down into a narrow and steep dirt path. Our pace slowed dramatically as our heart rates picked up steam. Every few feet we would give each other a thumbs up to say, 'I'm okay—let's keep going! Onward and upward!'

"Under my breath I was saying *Geeeesh, this is starting to kick me in the pants!*

"And that's where we found her."

"Who? *Who* did you find?" Emily interrupted, sure that the "who" was a famous celebrity.

"We were startled to find this sweet woman who appeared to around 40ish, leaning against a rock, breathing heavy and fanning herself. We immediately stopped, offered water, and asked if we could help. Between breaths she assured us that she was okay and just needed a slower pace than the group she was with. She managed a half-smile trying to reassure us she was fine."

"And that's exactly why I stay on the veranda of my hotel," Emily said, emphatically.

"After a few minutes, her breathing returned to normal and she appeared to be fully recovered. We found out her name was Elizabeth, and she and her group of friends from Iowa had been planning this trip to Hawaii for several months. Climbing Diamond Head was at the top of their bucket list. We asked Elizabeth if she wanted us to accompany her the rest of the way up so she could see the top but she politely declined.

"Oh no, you guys go ahead. I'm fine, really. I guess I thought it wasn't..." Elizabeth's voice started to crack.

She composed her emotions but couldn't hide her disappointment. "It just seemed so easy at the bottom. Someone should post a warning sign down there and let people know that it doesn't finish the way it starts! I had no idea it was going to become so steep. I guess I won't see the top this time but I sent my camera on up with my friends. They'll take plenty of pictures for me.

"I thought I'd be okay, you know," Elizabeth added, quietly. She tried her best to fight back emotion as she reached down to grab her back pack and slipped it over her shoulders.

"Hey, thanks for stopping to check on me. That was so nice of you guys. I'll just wait for my friends at the bottom." And she turned to head back down the trail.

"Well that is just so sad," Emily said with concern. "I feel bad for Elizabeth and I don't even know her."

"I know. We felt terrible for her as well. Who wouldn't? She was going to miss an unforgettable, mountaintop experience that she had planned for months! Disappointment was written all over her face but she tried to hide it as she headed back.

"Mike and I stood there a little stunned by what had just happened and slowly made our way to the top. As I stood at the pinnacle of that extinct volcano and admired the splendor, I couldn't stop thinking about Elizabeth. *Was she okay? Was someone at the bottom comforting her as she waited for her friends? Were there others that had to turn back as well?* It broke my heart. Even if her friends were professional photographers, they couldn't capture the overwhelming beauty held in that special moment. She had missed a once-in-a-lifetime opportunity with her friends during her magical trip that could never be replaced and my heart was broken for her."

"Sounds like you did everything you could to help her," Emily said, trying to console me.

"I did one more thing for her that I know helps more than anything—I prayed."

"How did you pray for her? Did she hear you?"

"No, I just prayed in my heart that God would help her never miss another mountaintop."

Emily nodded her head, and added, "I'm gonna add an Amen to that."

Emily paused and confessed, "Truth be told, I've wanted to climb Diamond Head for a long time—years, really. I don't want to only see it from the veranda. I guess in some ways I've always been afraid I would end up like Elizabeth. Embarrassed. Heartbroken. And defeated."

"Emily, you don't have to see Diamond Head from a distance. That is the entire point of this story. You can climb that mountain, or *any* mountain, if you will do two things: set your mind to it and prepare for it. That is all it takes. Decide and prepare. And how do we prepare? That's the power of exercise. It helps us find inspiration and courage as it strengthens and emboldens our entire body, mind, and soul. Once you start to see results in your stamina and strength, you'll be able to set your mind on other dreams you once thought were too big! And that will put a fire in your belly to overcome the greatest mountains in your life! Now doesn't that sound better than sitting on a veranda just *looking* at Diamond Head? You can stand on top of it and pump your fist in victory!"

"Laurie, I never thought I would say this but that *is* what I want! Don't get me wrong—I love lounging on my veranda. But I also want to experience more of life. I need to stop sitting back scared out of my wits that I can't do something. What am I so flippin' afraid of? I'm tired of it holding me back from really living!"

I could hear a new resolve in Emily's voice as she continued, "I didn't get where I am today in my career because I let obstacles get in the way. And I'm sure the heck not going to let it steal my other dreams—especially in Hawaii!"

"That's the spirit, Emily! This is exactly why exercise matters. You don't want to miss out on a beautiful mountain in Hawaii or anything else you set your mind to and prepare for. Your energy and strength can help you accomplish it! You just need them to cooperate."

"So how do I get them to cooperate? 'Cause right now they feel like rebels. "

"You train them by doing the things that are hard. You tell your energy and strength where and when they are going to work. They do not tell you. Stop letting them off the hook. They are robbing you of an investment that will pay exponential dividends. You can accomplish what you decide and prepare for, Emily! I know you can if you want it enough and you're willing to step forward in courage. What do ya say, Em? Do I see a hike to Diamond Head in your future?" I asked, hoping against all odds.

"Yes you do! And Jeffrey is going to be right beside me. No more sitting on the sidelines for this girl. I need to stop thinking my health is good enough. That I won't be the one to miss mountaintops, when I know in my heart of hearts that I'm in the same boat as Elizabeth. I just never wanted to admit it." Emily declared.

"You know, Em, I used to say to myself *'I'm really okay. I may not be in tip-top shape, but there's no way I'm as bad off as some other people I know.'* But that kept me from becoming my best me. That kind of ordinary thinking is what keeps us from climbing magnificent mountains and believing all of our dreams are within reach."

"I have heard people say that—and I think I've said it myself," Emily admitted.

"The problem is that it *is* incredibly easy to identify people worse off. Just look around and you will see plenty of unhealthy people. If we compare ourselves to the worst of them we will always come out looking like a poster child of health. A diseased body will eventually accompany our lack of exercise. Unfortunately it often requires a medical emergency for folks to wake up to the reality that exercise can, not just get them up a mountain, but actually save their lives.

"My aha moment was my hair falling out. I knew that was a reflection of the damage going on inside of me from stress. A lot of people wait for that moment of desperation before they turn to the habits that could actually help *prevent* many diseases."

"I'm not going to wait for a crisis to get healthy, Laurie! I'd rather prevent disease any day than treat it."

"It truly is so much easier to prevent than treat. Heart disease, in particular, is shockingly prevalent in our society these days. Recently, Dr. John Warner, 52, President of the American Heart Association, suffered a heart attack less than 24 hours after speaking at a medical conference! He said he felt fine that morning but just a short time later in his hotel room his heart stopped completely! His daughter began

CPR and a doctor and nurse at the hotel used a defibrillator to restart his heart! They saved his life! Dr. Warner said he had no symptoms. All of a sudden, he just collapsed!"

"Oh my goodness! If it can happen to Dr. Warner, it can happen to any of us!"

"That's right, Em. Dr. Warner had no warning signs even though heart disease was obviously present.

"Even Bob Harper, the famous *Biggest Loser* personal trainer, suffered a massive heart attack in 2017 at the age of 51! Bob attributed his heart attack to stress, lack of rest, and genetics. He had stopped breathing and was turning blue, according to his book *The Super Carb Diet,* but a doctor happened to be in the gym with him and gave him life-saving CPR. They called his heart attack the Widow maker because it is so often fatal."

"Holy cow!! *Bob Harper*??"

"And yet, so many people think it could never happen to them— because it hasn't *yet.*

"Here's a statistic I find shocking. The *American Heart Association* has been telling us for years that heart disease is the number killer in America with *one out of three people dying from it!* That doesn't even take into consideration those who suffer from its effects with a decreased quality of life while still living."

"Wow, one out of three people *die* from heart disease?" Emily asked. "That's an astonishing number. I had no idea heart disease affected that many people."

"To put that significant number into perspective, when I speak on this topic, I have people think of 2 friends they know and love. Then I ask, 'Which 1 of the 3 of you do you think will die from heart disease?' The answer is always the same, 'None of us!'

"Somehow people don't fear it could ever happen to them or those they love even though statistics prove time and time again that their chance of dying from heart disease, at a 1-out-of-3 ratio, is very real. That blows my mind and grieves my heart.

"Turns out, according to the Chapman University study on what Americans most fear, it appears that people are more afraid of reptiles, tornadoes, and heights,[1] then they are from what is a bazillion times more apt to take them out! Dying of heart disease didn't even make the list! I have a very difficult time accepting the fact that, in spite of all of the education, public service announcements, and constant research imploring us to fight heart disease by living healthier lifestyles, many people still don't believe it can happen to them."

"I think I've been in denial most of my life about these very issues."

"I was abruptly yanked out of denial at 19 when my dad suffered his third heart attack and tragically passed away at only 52 years of age. Since then I've lost both of my husband's parents, as well as countless friends, to this horrific and epidemic disease. And the numbers are getting worse. Heart disease is no longer an *old-person's disease*. I've lost friends in their thirties to heart attacks who had no clue that disease, let alone death, was imminent."

"I'm so sorry about your daddy, Laurie," Emily said softly as she touched my shoulder. "I've lost loved ones to heart disease as well and it is heart-breaking."

"Thank you, Emily. I've lived my entire adult life without my dad and it is a deep, tragic loss. That's one of the reasons I'm so committed to helping others understand—there's a lot of living to do so let's do what we can to keep a largely preventable disease from stealing our dreams and future."

"I can understand that. I'm concerned that heart disease seems to run in my family. Is there anything I can do to protect myself?"

"The first thing you can do is look at your risk of heart disease. As I explain the factors, see if any of them apply to you. While the first two risk factors are impossible to change, it is possible to improve the others. The first factor is age. The older you are the greater the chances of developing heart disease since it can begin in childhood. This is a very important reason why children should be playing outside or in a gym instead of *sitting* for recreation. There's enough of that in adulthood.

"The second factor is gender. Men have a greater propensity to have heart attacks at a younger age since estrogen is found to have some protective properties. After menopause, however, the ratios are equal.

"The third factor is genetics. Unfortunately it's impossible to change your DNA. However, recent studies confirm that implementing a healthy lifestyle earlier in life can help counter it. Two large studies from *Northwestern Medicine* confirm that a healthy lifestyle has the biggest impact on cardiovascular health. One study shows the majority of people who adopted healthy lifestyle behaviors in young adulthood maintained a low cardiovascular risk profile in middle age. The other study shows cardiovascular health is due primarily to lifestyle factors and healthy behavior.

"According to Donald Lloyd-Jones, M.D., chair and professor of preventive medicine at *Northwestern University Feinberg School of Medicine* and a staff cardiologist at Northwestern Memorial Hospital. 'Health behaviors can trump a lot of your genetics.'[2] This research shows that people have a level of control over their heart health. The earlier they start making healthy choices, the more likely they are to maintain a low-risk profile for heart disease."

"Wow, so there is hope for me even though I have family members with heart disease. That is good news and certainly a reason to try to prevent heart disease. There are just so many constraints it puts on a person's abilities and quality of life. What else should I be watching for?"

"The fourth indicator is smoking. Smoking is one of the worst habits ever because it causes such rapid decline in your health! Smokers between the ages of 35 and 70 have death rates *3 times higher* than those who have never smoked! Unfortunately, I know this one all too well since my dad smoked more than a pack a day.

"A friend of mine who is a radiologist tells me every time I see him, 'Tell people not to smoke, Laurie! It is an insidious disease and one of the worst things you can do to your body! It makes for a terrible life and a horrible death.'"

Emily was moved to tears, "Laurie, you've *got* to talk to Jeffrey. Please. Help him kick his addiction. I can't even imagine going through the rest of my life without him or seeing him suffer. *Please.*"

I put my arm around Emily's shoulder. "Absolutely! I will do everything in my power to help Jeffrey stop smoking. There are some very effective cessation programs out there that have had wonderful results. I'll let him know what those are and he can sign up when he's ready. Does that sound like a plan?"

Emily nodded, smiling slightly and wiping her eyes. "That sounds like a good plan. Thank you. I want to hear more. What else can we do to avoid heart disease?"

"The fifth factor is a sedentary lifestyle and obesity. With the rise of electronic technology and conveniences at every turn, people don't move as much as they did even a generation ago. The more you sit, the more obesity threatens your health. The statistics in America are staggering—7 out of 10 people are overweight and out of those 7, every 3 are obese."

"Oh my goodness, I sit all day long!" Emily exclaimed.

"But you've already started walking every day so you're on your way to getting healthier," I said, reassuringly. "Let's celebrate what you're doing right because when you consider all of the changes you have already made, it is a one-two punch against heart disease."

"Yeah, let's celebrate all the good—but I still want to know everything I can."

I continued with the sixth risk factor, "Hypertension—high blood pressure is extremely dangerous since it damages blood vessel walls and organs. It's often called the silent killer since you don't see its profound damage until it's often too late. When pressure is high, the force of the blood through your arteries and blood vessels can be compared to watering your garden with a fire hose. High blood pressure often causes irreparable damage to your blood vessels. That's why it can be life-threatening."

I had Emily's undivided attention. "High cholesterol is the seventh risk factor. Your body makes all the cholesterol you need. Any excess is deposited in your blood vessels and that can create a blockage which often requires a surgical stent or even open heart surgery to correct it. The surgery may allow healthy blood-flow to return to the heart and the rest of your body, but it is not without major risks."

"And lastly, the eighth risk factor is stress. While everyone handles stress differently, the greatest correlation of stress to heart disease, according to the *American Heart Association*, occurs when it causes coping mechanism behaviors like smoking, drinking, overeating, or physical inactivity. Those habits only exacerbate the threat of developing heart disease by increasing obesity, high blood pressure, and cholesterol levels.[3]

Stress also disrupts gut health which is command central for health throughout the rest of your body. When the bacteria microbiome is out of balance—and stress easily damages the good bacteria—we now know that Dysbiosis (more bad than good gut bacteria) will increase inflammation throughout the body and exacerbate some of the risk factors like high blood pressure, high cholesterol, and obesity. Emily counted up her risk factors and showed me on her fingers, "I have 4 risk factors. Oh my word! I was hoping I wouldn't have *any*! What can I do to improve them?"

I raised an eyebrow, and Emily smiled knowingly. We both answered simultaneously, "Exercise!"

"Because the heart is a muscle, Emily, it can be strengthened by exercise, and aerobic exercise specifically has a huge benefit to the heart. An expert panel, gathered by the *U.S. Department of Health and Human Services*, found that regular physical activity can cut the risk of heart attacks and strokes by at least 20 percent and reduce the chance of early death.[4] A strong heart makes the rest of the body work more efficiently.

"Honestly, Emily, exercise is another tool that can change your life!

"The first day we met, you told me that you wanted to 'stop feeling awful and get some flippin' energy?' Do you remember?"

"Yes, of course. I've been saying that for years. I've just been afraid of what it would take to get healthy." Emily admitted with surprising candor. "You knew my sarcasm and saltiness were just a front for my fears. But I'm sick and tired of being sick and tired! Enough is enough. I'm ready to do whatever it takes and if exercise is one of the tools I need then so be it! I'm ready for more."

"And more you shall receive!" I responded, smiling. "Exercise is the key to getting more of what you want—more stamina, more energy, more strength, more weight loss, more confidence, more ability to relentlessly pursue your goals and dreams, and that makes for a more extraordinary life.

"Listen to this little tidbit. When you exercise, your body manufactures more red blood cells. The red blood cells carry iron and iron carries oxygen. That means the more red blood cells you create, the more energy you feel!"

Emily was absorbing the information like a sponge and nodding her head in agreement.

"In a study published in the planner *Psychotherapy and Psychosomatics* in 2008, *University of Georgia* researchers found that inactive folks who normally complained of fatigue could increase energy by 20% while decreasing fatigue by as much as 65% by simply participating in regular, low-intensity exercise.[5] Some of that energy comes from the foods you consume, and is also affected by water and sleep, as we've discussed previously. You also have little powerhouses inside your muscles called mitochondria that produce more energy as you increase exercise."

I explained, "For the first time, Americans are raising children who may grow up less healthy than their parents. Many kids are more inactive than adults, preferring to play videogames and engage in online social networking instead of moving their bodies with exercise. When fatigue can no longer be blamed on winter hibernation, the cure may be as simple as starting to move, even if it's the last thing you feel like doing."

I wanted Emily to understand that even a little exercise was better than none, "Researchers at the *University of Georgia* found that sedentary, otherwise healthy adults who engaged in as little as 20 minutes of low-to-moderate aerobic exercise, 3 days a week for 6 consecutive weeks, reported feeling less fatigued and more energized. While fatigue can be a symptom of various health problems, including serious conditions such as heart disease and cancer, research has reportedly shown that 1 in 4 people suffer from general fatigue that isn't due to a known medical condition."[6]

Pete McCall, Exercise Physiologist at the *American Council on Exercise* said, "If a sedentary individual begins an exercise program it will enhance the blood flow carrying oxygen and nutrients to muscle tissue improving their ability to produce more energy."[7]

Emily was intrigued that exercise could improve so many areas where she had been struggling.

"Exercise also reduces stress! It's the only behavior that uses up surplus adrenaline that's released when you face a stressful situation, and provides mood-lifting hormones like endorphins that promote a sense of calm and well-being. If exercise were available as a pill, experts say, everyone would be taking it since exercise is so good at defusing stress. This creates a cyclic effect since reduced stress also helps you sleep better. And when you sleep better, you have more emotional reserves to handle the problems that create stress in the first place. Researchers confirm there is a very strong link between regular exercise and improved emotions. Other coping behaviors like eating, smoking, and drinking may give the illusion of providing relief and comfort, but they only exacerbate the problems and end up creating additional stresses.

"I know firsthand that kind of coping behavior is an oxymoron. It promises peace but furnishes pain. Exercise, however…"

"Helps us conquer mountains!" Emily interjected.

"Right, Em!"

"With all my bedtime rituals now—and prayer—my stress, while not completely gone, is way more manageable."

I congratulated Emily on her progress. "Look at you, girlfriend! You've made a significant shift in your commitment to change and now you're already reaping some benefits. That will help perpetuate your momentum as you embrace even more change."

"More change? You're back to exercise, aren't you?"

"Yes, ma'am," I responded, laughing. "There are still more advantages to be gained from exercise. It increases good HDL (high density lipoprotein) cholesterol and decreases bad LDL (low density lipoprotein)."

"Okay, I've heard of those. I'm just not sure what they are."

"Here's an analogy that might help you understand. Have you ever lived with a messy roommate? LDL cholesterol is like a bad roommate that leaves *stuff* everywhere. In this case, the *stuff* is waxy fat, also known as bad cholesterol that sticks to blood vessels, severely damaging them. HDL cholesterol is very important to your health since it acts as the organized roommate, picking up all the messes that LDLs leave behind. Just remember, messy is bad, as in lethal. And clean is good, as in life-saving. Exercise gives you more of the good in HDL, less of the bad in LDL."

"Yes, I want more of the good! I always appreciated an organized roomie and that's exactly what I want in my cholesterol."

"As if that weren't enough, exercise also creates collateral circulation. People who exercise on a regular basis can actually manufacture additional blood vessels! If there would happen to be a blockage in your blood vessels from plaque buildup that prevented your blood from getting through the main arteries, the *new* collateral circulation could create a detour so the blood can get through to the rest of the body to keep you alive. And of course, the more fit you are, the more detours you can build which increases your chance of surviving a traumatic heart episode.

"Exercise also reduces your risk of developing type 2 diabetes. In the federal *Diabetes Prevention Program*, modest lifestyle changes, like regular exercise, delayed or prevented the onset of type 2 diabetes by 58%—a better rate than that achieved with the diabetes drug metformin."[8]

I concluded the list by explaining to Emily, "And finally, last but not least, weight loss is a wonderful benefit of exercise. One of the key ingredients to losing body fat is exercise since it raises your metabolism, the rate at which you use up calories. It's more than just burning excess calories—it changes you from the inside out to make you leaner. Without it, your body can dig in its heels to work against you and hang on to fat."

I continued by confessing, "I struggled with my metabolism for months after my divorce! I tried to lose weight without exercise at first. No matter how far I reduced my calories, I got to the point where I couldn't lose weight because my metabolism was so low. I was starving myself, then bingeing because I was starving! I was so frustrated! I felt enslaved to the idea that cutting calories would make me lose weight. And when it didn't, I felt the shackles of shame tighten their grip, which perpetuated the cycle of starving and bingeing again and again. And that, my friend, is a recipe for how to gain weight."

Emily looked incredulous, and replied, "No one would ever guess that about you, Laurie."

"Healing in my heart brought the real transformation I needed for healing in my body. That was the first step. Then losing weight started by taking control of my metabolism. And do you know how I did that, Emily?"

"I bet you're going to say exercise," Emily answered.

"You bet I am! I eventually broke through those roadblocks and got my metabolism back on track because of exercise. One of the reasons it's so life-changing is because it changes your body chemically on the inside first before results ever show on the outside. When you exercise, you develop more enzymes that work to help release fat for energy! The same is true if you are sedentary and don't exercise—you develop enzymes that actually promote fat storage and keep you fatter!

"In addition to creating important enzymes that actually work to facilitate using fat for energy, aerobic exercise also as the ability to put a psychological brake on how much you eat. When you work aerobically, your body likes to use fat for energy instead of sugar in your bloodstream, and that seems to shut off the switch for hunger. It also creates more Leptin—the hormone that shuts down appetite. When you realize that 20 minutes on the elliptical only burns about 150 calories, you start to think twice about eating anything extra because you understand how hard it is to work it off.

"Anything that improves your quality of life and can even extend your life is worth doing. Aerobic exercise is a super-hero that can accomplish both of those," I said enthusiastically.

"I want some of those fat-releasing enzymes!" Emily exclaimed. "I didn't even know they existed. That certainly adds a new twist to aerobic exercise—making my body work for me and not against me for once. Love that one."

Now that Emily was sold on aerobic exercise it was time to tackle the importance of strength training and hope she would buy in to that idea as well.

"Another form of exercise that promotes good health, reduces the risk of developing many diseases, and helps you live a longer and healthier life is strength training."

Emily tried to muffle a groan.

"I heard that," I replied, "and it is not going to deter me from adding it to your plan. I promise you it works."

Emily protested. "But I'm already doing a ton of work—drinking about 80 ounces of water daily and keeping my special cup with me, sleeping longer and better with all my bedtime rituals—oh yeah, and we got a new mattress that is dreamy—plus I'm shutting down my iPad early, making lists of what I'm thankful for, and praying every night. Doesn't that earn me any credit?"

"Of course it does," I responded. "But let me ask you this. Do you feel tons better, have more energy, and find that you are able to sleep through the night now?"

"Absolutely! I would have to say yes to all three."

"Then I think you can probably trust that I'm not going to have you waste time on anything that doesn't work, right?"

"Yeah, I guess so," Emily admitted, still resisting. "I am just not very strong. Or disciplined. Never really have been. And that makes it seem harder than it is, I guess."

"In our next session we'll talk about all the ways you can make exercise fun—even for strength. There are so many options now to train your body. Lifting weights is not just for athletes or power lifters—or guys. The benefits of strength training far exceed muscle development. It is a powerful way to boost your metabolism and make your muscles, joints, and bones dramatically stronger. And that is no small thing."

Emily still wasn't completely sold on the idea so I shared a list of additional benefits to further sway her.

"Strength training makes it easier to lose weight. Muscles use a ton of calories so you're less likely to become overweight or obese. According to Dr. Lee, Professor of medicine at Harvard Medical School, 'The more muscle you have, the more calories you burn, so it's easier to maintain your weight. Muscles are helping you lose weight even while you are sleeping!'"[9]

"While I *sleep*? That's fantastic!" Emily said, clapping her hands.

I loved Emily's enthusiasm. "Not only that, exercise makes you more protected from diseases like arthritis and osteoporosis. It can even relieve stress on your heart. Muscles that are consistently worked make handling daily chores less of a strain, which buffers the workload on the heart.

"Unfortunately, no matter how hard you work at keeping your muscles strong, you start to lose conditioning in a very short amount of time. It only takes 3 days of not working out before we begin to experience *deconditioning* in our bodies. On the average, a somewhat sedentary man who hasn't maintained regular lifting workouts in his mid-forties has already lost between 10 and 14 pounds of muscle, compared to a man in his mid-twenties. As muscle tissue decreases, your body uses fewer calories. A pound of fat needs only 2 calories a day to maintain itself. A pound of muscle needs an astonishing 35 to 40 calories!"

Emily raised her eyebrows. "So, you're saying I will need *more* food if I have more muscle? That seems like a wonderful benefit!"

"Exactly. That's the power of having a revved up metabolism."

"Well, let's get to revving! Time's a wastin'!"

"I'm glad you're onboard, Emily. Strength-training has been such an important road to my recovery. Even in my fifties, I find that it adds significant benefit to my energy. It really has value for every adult, and can be profoundly helpful as we age. Once a person reaches their 50s and beyond, strength or resistance training is critical to preserving the ability to perform the most ordinary activities of daily living—like carrying groceries or climbing stairs."

"Or hiking Diamond Head!" Emily added.

"Absolutely. The stronger you are, the smaller mountains become."

"Strength comes from optimal exercise that includes both aerobics and weight lifting. 'Just doing aerobic exercise is not adequate,' says Dr. Robert Schreiber, physician-in-chief at *Hebrew Senior Life* and an instructor in medicine at *Harvard Medical School*.[10] Unless you are doing strength training, you *will* become weaker and less functional." I explained.

"All right, I'm sold," Emily said with reluctant resolve.

"Okay, good, because we have one last piece of exercise to add and that is stretching. Most clients I train seem to be far less concerned initially with their stretching than they are with other aspects of exercise. I guess they feel it doesn't accomplish much, but once they start doing it they learn very quickly how important it is. Stretching often takes a backseat to aerobic exercise or strength training because we can't always see its results. And most people are in a huge time crunch so stretching gets left out. But it is truly very important to our health. We've known for decades that stretching can help prevent injuries, increase circulation, keep muscles working more effectively, improve flexibility and joint range of motion, and improve performance. The problem is that there are too many mixed messages about *when* to stretch, *how to* stretch, *how long* to hold a stretch, and *how often* to stretch. Do I stretch before or after working out? Do I need to stretch every day even if I don't work out? Is stretching a good warm-up?"

"Yes, I've wondered all those questions too."

"Here are a few things to remember about stretching. First, don't try to stretch cold muscles. They can tear unless they're pliable. And they become pliable by warming up first. Always start with some gentle movements that involve your large lower body muscles to gradually get your blood pumping and raise your core temperature. Walk or run for 10 minutes or so, use the elliptical, bike, whatever you want that gets you moving and feeling warmer. Once you feel warm that's a good indication that your muscles are ready to stretch. Think of your muscles like taffy. When taffy is cold it's resistant to stretching. But once heat is applied to it, it becomes loose and pliable."

"Next, always stretch a muscle *after* an activity. Using a muscle requires it to contract and release, contract and release, which shortens it. To keep good flexibility you want to elongate that muscle back out by holding a stretch for about 20 seconds. Then relax. Stretch it again and hold. Then relax. Also, never bounce into a stretch. Hold it again a little deeper into the muscle each time."

"I think I've got it," Emily announced proudly. "Aerobic exercise. Strength train. Stretch. When do we start?"

"How about right now? Let's jump into our next discussion on how we make all this happen."

"You know, I'm actually looking forward to it!" Emily admitted. "Never thought I'd say that. Man! I'm gonna conquer this exercise thing! And who knows what else!"

Good thing because Hawaii is calling. And not from a veranda.

Chapter 6
Do What You Love—It Will Love You Back

Emily quickly settled in after her bathroom break and I noticed she had also refilled her water bottle.

Such remarkable progress.

"Fantastic, by the way," I said, grinning.

"What?" Emily asked, sarcastically. "You mean my water consumption or my blazing speed?"

"Well, both actually. Now that you mention it, you do have a little spring in your step."

Emily smiled widely, "I love it! I woke up this morning without an alarm for the first time in years. And I actually feel energized. Who would have thought that drinking more water and getting some great sleep would make me feel so much better?" Emily paused as she rolled her eyes, "Well, besides *you* of course?"

"You're funny, Em. More and more people are discovering that good health doesn't have to be complicated. What makes you feel different is right inside here," I said pointing to Emily's heart, "and when your heart and head agree to work together that is what makes you new from the inside out!.

"Things in me are definitely changing, slowly but surely. I feel a little better each day

"I can't tell you how happy that makes me. You're working so hard to be consistent with your first two tools and that is the pathway toward achieving all your goals. One perpetuates the next.

"Today I'm going to add some other exercise strategies for you to consider as well. Sound good?"

"Yep," Emily responded. "I'm ready for options. What do you have, Teach?"

Wow, this was a side of Emily that had drastically changed from the first day—no fear, just confidence and excitement for embracing new challenges. Her energy was soaring and her positive outlook was almost palpable. I was so happy for her and the tremendous progress she was making. We had come a long way in a short time, but there was still an ominous road in front of us.

"Let's talk about the 5 most frequently asked exercise questions clients have for me."

"Yes! I bet I have the same ones!"

"The first question clients seem to always ask about exercising is usually something like 'How hard should I be exercising?' That's really a question about intensity."

"Yeah, I've always wondered that as well, Laurie. How do I know what level is right for me? And what's the most effective range of intensity?"

"There's a very simple test you can employ called *The Talk Test*. It works like this: aerobic means *with air* so an effective aerobic exercise will promote the use and supply of *extra* oxygen. You should be working strenuously enough that you need your mouth open for air. But not so intensely that you can't carry on a conversation. You should feel the need to take a breath about every 4 or 5 words with no gasping. That means a leisurely stroll through the park where you can converse at the same comfort level as when you are sitting down indicates you need to work harder. Strolling as you walk is *movement*, which is always better than sitting. However, it does not qualify as *aerobic* unless you increase your breathing. Conversely, a 30 second sprint that completely takes your breath away is not what I'm talking about either. There's nothing wrong with sprinting—it's just not sustainable for everyone."

"Well thank goodness for that because there's no way sprinting is happening here!" Emily retorted.

"The second question concerns frequency—how often should I exercise? You may have heard that 3 times a week is the goal to shoot for but my suggestion is for much more than that."

"Of course it is," Emily teased.

"I suggest exercising 5 to 6 days a week."

"Whoa! That seems like a lot, don't you think?"

If you only exercise 3 days out of a 7-day week you still have more days that you're *not* exercising. Do you sit at work daily? Do you have stress that you need to unload? Do your joints ache? Do you want more energy? Do you want to lose weight?" I asked.

"That would be "yes" to all four," Emily answered, with her thumbs up.

"Well, then daily aerobic exercise is the best way to remedy those issues," I said. "Plus, the everyday commitment seems to be another key component for success since it eliminates the decision-making that can derail even the best of intentions. If you give yourself the option of missing a workout, guess what? You will. It's amazing how much easier it is to miss the next time. And the next. Before you know it, a month goes by without exercising. That's not the direction you want to head."

"Nope, I've been down the roller-coaster of inconsistency and that is not a ride I want to be on any longer. I like where we're headed."

"So let's consider question three which is about duration, 'How long should I exercise?' The correct answer is 20-60 minutes. For most healthy individuals, the minimum time to exercise to achieve improvement or maintenance in cardiorespiratory fitness is 20 minutes. There may be days when it's tough to fit in even that. But remember, anything is better than nothing and if you only have 10 minutes then make it your best 10 minutes."

Emily nodded. "So just 20 minutes or more is preferable—10 or whatever I have is acceptable. Mouth open for air. Okay, that seems doable; I may even start walking faster and up my intensity a bit."

"Now you're talking, Emily. Every little bit of progress leads you toward bigger changes in your energy levels and your overall health! I love what I'm hearing."

"I knew you would. I'm not crazy like you yet but I'm working on it. I mean that with love, by the way," Emily said, smiling.

Music to my ears, by the way.

"Another frequently asked question I hear is 'how can I stay motivated?' And I believe the best answer is to have fun, make it feel like *play*, and don't do the same exercise every day. Change it up. I don't care how much a person loves running or circuit training or TRX or cycling, their muscles will remember what they did the last time they worked out. It will become progressively easier. Muscle memory is a real phenomenon, hence the term, *it's just like riding a bike.* Your muscles remember. Plus, the same movement can get boring very quickly. Both your muscles and your brain greatly benefit from changing up one or more factors.

"For committed runners I always suggest trying new trails, joining a running club, or doing occasional races for charity. For *Zumba* fans, I suggest trying different instructors or routines.

"I'm seeing a lot of creativity in the fitness world right now so change it up. I've even seen a surfboard workout in a pool that looks amazingly fun."

"Surfboard??What in the world?!!"

"We just need to find the right activity for you, Emily, that's both challenging and fun. And prepares you for Diamond Head. I know you've been walking for exercise. Do you love it yet?"

"I wouldn't exactly use the word *love.*"

"So maybe to add some interest, you could ask some friends to join you and try different trails. Walking is an excellent choice as an initial foray into exercise. It's been said that walking may be one of the most powerful *medicines* available since it's convenient, free, and makes a great impact on your energy and health

"But I do think you would enjoy branching out a bit as well. I'd also like to see you try some spinning classes or find a beautiful park to ride your bike in—and you can always add a hill or two.

"Even better, rework your routine completely. Cycle one week, walk hills the next, take a dance class the week after that, try some Pilates or whatever keeps you excited for the next workout. Muscle confusion gives you a more effective workout and keeps your brain interested. But above all, trying new activities should feel like play and be enjoyable enough to keep you coming back for more. "

"How about a *Hula Hoop*?" Emily asked, with a twinge of sarcasm. "Can I exercise effectively doing that? I used to be the neighborhood champ when I was a kid."

"Sure," I replied, smiling. "That sounds like a blast. Remember when you were growing up and your mom would say, 'Get outside and play?' Do that. Without a window in your office the sunshine would be good medicine, both emotionally and physically. Do something that is such a blast you can't wait to do it again! I think it's a double bonus if you can also find an activity to enjoy with your friends. Anything that promotes fun is a win-win!

"Other movement options can include tennis, especially singles tennis. Cycling is a great outdoor activity which is easy on your joints since there's little to no impact. Make sure you wear a helmet.

My goal was to give Emily plenty of variety so I added to the list, "Running is great aerobic exercise. You can enter a race that's a fundraiser. Run for a great cause and help get donations for the charity of your choice while you get fit. It will make those miles even more meaningful to you and beneficial to those in need."

"My running days are over. I know you'll find this shocking but I've always hated it. And I mean *hated* it!"

"Yep, I get it. There are too many options to do one you hate and you can do all the same fundraisers walking instead of running," I reminded her.

"Okay, great! Exercise and help a charity at the same time. I really like that."

"Hiking is also great exercise—truly one of my favorites! You get to enjoy the beauty and sounds of creation while you combine walking with climbing. Emily, we're fortunate enough to live in Tennessee where the hills are rolling and you can find amazing waterfalls in some of the nearby parks. And remember, Diamond Head is now a goal for you so hiking will help you train!"

"That's right," Emily remembered. "I guess you're not going to let me forget that one, are you?"

"Not a chance. It's a fantastic goal and I'm going to do my best to see that you accomplish it."

"Another wonderful outdoor exercise is skiing. It lets you enjoy the beauty of nature whether you're on a mountain, in the snow, or on a lake in the summer. Skiing is a great whole body activity that focuses on large muscles and balance, and anytime you can work on balance it's a bonus.

"I'll never forget seeing my sixty-year-old friend water-skiing on his heels without skis! He had so much fun! It was like watching a 10-year-old daredevil skiing with gray hair!

"Think about the way you used to play when you were young and see if going back to that doesn't spark some excitement and awaken some new courage as well. I grew up playing badminton and have recently found it again—what a trip back in time! Besides *Hula-hoop*, what were some of your favorites as a kid? What about *Frisbee*? Or soccer, basketball, jumping rope, paddle boarding, rock-climbing?"

"Before we started training together I would have rolled my eyes at all of those ideas, except *Hula-hoop* of course," Emily admitted. "But I also never thought I would be sleeping 7 hours straight, so—I guess—never say never. Although I don't see myself jumping rope now, I was the double-dutch queen, as well as the *Hula Hoop* champion back in the day. Maybe I could talk my friends into trying it again—at a much slower pace, of course. And paddle boarding—there's no reason why I can't learn how to do that in Waikiki—even at my age. I see people older than me trying it. Next time I'm in Hawaii it will be a very different trip."

That a girl, Emily! Your heart and head are cooperating and flexing a big muscle of courage. You're starting to sound unstoppable.

"For the days you can't get outside, how about trying a dance class? Dancing is a fun way to express yourself. It's all about enjoying the flow of the music and moving your body in a way you wouldn't normally move."

Emily chuckled, responding, "The only movement that is *normal* for my body is *sitting*. It probably wouldn't be pretty but it might just be a lot of fun, so yeah, why not?

"Group exercise classes like Orange Theory, Iron Tribe, TRX, and other circuit training classes have gained in popularity, and for good reason. They're challenging but the class is set up so everyone encourages you to keep working, keep pushing, keep doing the hard things. I just love that kind of class."

"Mmm, maybe I'll work up to that."

Okay, she didn't close the door completely. That was huge progress.

"There are also elliptical machines or swimming. These are both easy on the joints but very challenging. There's also racquetball, which is a fantastic workout and one that my husband and I still enjoy together. I doubt we'll ever stop playing since it was our first date 34 some years ago!"

"Aww, that is sweet—and a little strange," Emily said half-serious, half-teasing. "I mean, who has a first date *exercising*? You're supposed to have a romantic dinner, hold hands, and look into each other's eyes."

"We got to that eventually, but racquetball came first."

Emily laughed and shook her head. "I'd say you were out of your mind but 33 years in a happy marriage speaks for itself."

"It does indeed."

"Okay," Emily said, "Those are quite a few new ideas for movement. You make them all sound so worthwhile I don't know which one to try first!"

"And that, my friend is a great problem to have.

"The last question I seem to answer frequently for clients is "with all this new movement, what is the best way to protect against injury?"

"I would say, 'stay on my couch' but I'll bet that's not the right answer," Emily joked.

"Nope, not the couch. The answer is to wear high-quality athletic shoes."

"That was going to be my second answer," Emily retorted.

"As it turns out, shoes are a very big deal. This is one of the biggest mistakes I see clients make. They waste their money on the wrong shoes. "Trust me, I've seen it so many times I've lost track. Don't buy shoes that are *stylish* but don't offer excellent support. You'll end up paying for an expensive injury instead. You need a quality shoe that fits you perfectly to protect your feet and joints. If you end up injured, you could be paying a doctor bill instead.

"If you consider the fact that your feet absorb a shock that is twice the amount of your body weight when you walk, and FOUR times your body weight when you run, you'll want to ensure that you have the best shock absorbers possible! Whether you're walking, running, playing tennis, doing group exercise classes, or whatever activity you choose, start with shoes that fit you properly and have high-quality insoles— kind of like buying a good mattress. It does your body good."

"Absolutely worth the money and much cheaper than treating an injury. Could you relay this shoe information to Jeffrey as well? I think he's been using the same shoes for about 20 years. They don't last that long, do they?" Emily asked.

"Not unless they stay in your closet for 20 years without being worn," I teased. "The length of time athletic shoes last depends on the mileage you put on them. Elite athletes and marathon runners may have several pair of shoes at the same time so they can dry out the insoles between runs. The average person who walks or runs 4 to 5 times a week will probably need to replace their shoes twice a year. The best way to know is to try on new shoes in a store. If they feel different, you know you need new ones. I always use a good athletic shoe store like *Body 'n Sole*, where the salespeople can help me find just the right fit and make suggestions for any problems or pain I may be experiencing."

"Check. New shoes," Emily said, as she made an air check with her finger.

"One final component that needs to be added to your exercise routine is how to build your strength. This is different from aerobic conditioning in that you shouldn't work the same muscle group every day. After strength training, muscles need a 48-hour rest to recover completely. That's because when you lift weights you cause little micro tears in the muscle. If you pump your biceps on Monday, you should wait until Wednesday to do it again."

"Hang on just a sec, here," Emily interrupted. "You just said that lifting weights causes my muscles to tear. And I want that, why?"

"Because it makes the muscle stronger. The micro-tears initially break down the muscle but then after about 48 hours the muscle recovers and becomes stronger. That's why it takes a day of rest in between weight workouts. You can use machines or group strength classes or Pilates. Even YouTube and Instagram have some great videos that offer safe movements and helpful instruction. A couple of my Insty faves are jmarfit (Jennifer Martinez) and beautifullygracefullybroken (Tami Tyson). Everyone should always discuss their new exercise plan with their doctor and get their approval. Lucky for you, you're good to go!"

"Yay, lucky me." Emily responded sarcastically. "Okay, here's a question. Am I going to be sore? Because the thought of that is not appealing to me in the least bit. Not even remotely. Nada. Zip. Zero."

"I understand, Emily. Just know that a little muscle soreness in the beginning is normal. Not guaranteed, but it is a possibility.

"Lastly, don't forget to stretch! It really is so important and will help you increase your ability to move and protect yourself from injury. Remember to never bounce into a stretch. Just hold some tension on the muscle and keep it smooth."

"Boy, a lot has changed in 40 years. That was the only way we stretched in P.E.—bouncing to get a deeper stretch. Not so, huh?"

"Nope. Always hold your stretch. Breathe normally as you stretch. You should **go for tension, not pain.**"

"Alright. I appreciate this dialogue on the practical ways to include movement. It was a very thorough explanation of the benefits of aerobic conditioning, strength-training, and stretching. Wow, it can make such a difference in how we live, can't it? And yet I know so many people who never exercise. Heck, I was one of them! Why do you suppose that is?"

"Great question Emily. Bottom line is what we value we make time for. If it holds zero value to us we never get it on the calendar. If it does, we do. Simple. Harsh, maybe. But true. A lot of people feel they are too busy and they think they can't possibly squeeze one more thing into their day. But those are a cover-up for the real problem: it's just not important enough.

"I know it's cliché but everything worth having in life is worth fighting for. So while you may occasionally be slightly sore, you should remember that you will also be stronger, leaner, healthier, and more energetic with a body that works for you instead of against you. "

"What about the opposite kind of people, the ones who stay committed to exercise no matter how busy they get? Is that something you can teach me? Are there specific disciplines they use that keep them focused and on track?"

"Very insightful, Em! Fit people struggle too! No one is immune to the temptation of laziness, inconsistency, and lack of discipline. They just know how to overcome all of them.

"There are 3 habits they use to stay committed, even when they don't *feel* like it. The first is **enduring discomfort**. Navy SEALs call this *embracing the suck*. In his bestselling book, *The Way of the Seal*, U.S. Navy SEAL Commander Mark Divine explains the mental toughness required to lean into discomfort. 'When you consistently experience the personal growth that accrues from deliberately putting yourself out of balance, such as with challenging workouts, you begin to embrace temporary pain for the rewards it brings. The fear recedes into oblivion as you *embrace the suck*. The experience made me much stronger and wiser. There was nothing to fear from the pain.'[1]

"Emily, my clients who have experienced tremendous success with their fitness levels either instinctively knew or learned a new way to *embrace the suck*. Even if you only challenge yourself a little bit more each time, you will benefit in immeasurable ways both in the gym and in life, mentally and physically. You've already seen a difference in how you feel with just more water and sleep! Imagine how much stronger you're going to feel and how much more energy you will have by mastering this habit too—*embracing the suck*. If you want to make it to the top of Diamond Head you're going to have to learn this principle—be comfortable with discomfort."

"Number one, endure discomfort. I can't believe I'm saying this, but I will do my best! What else helps them succeed?"

"The second habit they use is **scheduling their workouts**, blocking the time as a very important appointment and guarding it against distractions. Are there emergencies that thwart even the best-laid plans and schedules? Of course! But people who are seriously committed to their exercise routine get right back to it as soon as possible. When you start to see significant improvements in how you feel, it provides powerful motivation to keep it scheduled and guard the next workout as you would a meeting with a VIP client. It's an inspiring and self-perpetuating cycle so guard that *appointment*. Don't allow yourself an "unexcused absence" because it can trigger continual absenteeism and perpetuate non-commitment. Then you're right back at square one."

"I've come too far to go back to square one. I will make sure my workouts are on my schedule as VIP appointments."

"The third habit that seems to help tremendously is being around a **network of supportive people**. You've got to receive an infusion of daily encouragement from your circle of friends or family to have the greatest success. Whether they workout with you or provide regular words of affirmation to steady your resolve, those with whom you surround yourself can make or break your results. Make sure their influence strengthens your commitment. And be proactive about avoiding people who try to sabotage your dedication because they feel bad about their own unhealthy decisions.

"You've no doubt heard the saying, *show me your friends and I'll show you your future*. It rings true for your exercise plan too. So make sure you choose a circle of friends that will ignite the fire of hope and commitment in you every day."

"I love that—a circle of fire. Didn't somebody sing about a circle of fire—or a ring of friends? Or something like that? I know I've heard it before."

"Johnny Cash sang *A Ring of Fire* and Point of Grace sang *Circle of Friends*. Two totally different messages," I mused.

"Oh, I knew I'd heard them before," Emily laughed.

"Speaking of different messages, next week we're going to discuss our final topic for your personal training. Yep, the one you've been waiting for with bated breath—FOOD! I absolutely cannot wait! It's going to be so empowering for you! I know you will love it."

"How can you say that?" Emily asked incredulously. "It will be the *worst* week ever! You're going to tell me all the stuff I can't eat! What could be empowering and exciting about that?" Emily grumbled.

"Everything! You'll see."

Emily groaned. "I'll be here but I will not be happy about it."

Doesn't matter—I've got enough happy for both of us. Girl, you got mountains to climb! And your Circle of Friends is going to help you get there.

Chapter 7
Food is Fuel

"I'm on a short leash today," Emily informed me as we met in the hallway to begin her final session. "I may have to leave a little early for meetings and such."

"Meetings?" I asked, surprised she hadn't mentioned that before our last week.

"Yep, *all* morning—starting early," Emily replied winking.

Okay, I get it. Not so fast there, Em.

"You know, I bet you will be pleasantly surprised that you'll actually like our conversation about food today. Here's a fresh spin for you—I'm not going to tell you what you *can't* eat."

"You're not? How is that possible?" she asked, surprised and a little confused.

"No, I'm not. That's not my job. My job is to present food options and explain how they help you. But then it's up to you to choose *what* you eat. There are guidelines for what we know works well in the body and what doesn't, but everyone is different. That final decision is yours. Just like you chose how much water to drink, how to prepare for sleep, and what kind of exercise to do, you will also decide how to feed your body."

"That sounds fair. Maybe I can be a minute or two late for my meetings."

"Perfect, Emily. For starters, let's take a walk back in time and look at how it used to be in the good 'ole days. Growing up in the Midwest in the sixties, mealtime for me was always simple, predictable, and delicious. We could count on meat, potatoes, and vegetables on our plates every night. My mom was a master at preparing a variety of that combo and really didn't deviate from it. Like ever. We never had dessert except for birthdays and holidays. If we were having a special dinner we would occasionally have fruit—usually berries—for dessert. Wild living, right?"

Emily laughed. "I grew up the same way. Uncanny."

"Dinner would always consist of meat from our local farmers with chicken, beef, and pork, and fish once a week from the market, combined with red or sweet potatoes that were mashed, boiled, or baked, topped off with vegetables from some neighbor's garden like beets, tomatoes, cucumbers, broccoli, green beans, peas, or carrots.

"I ate what was on my plate and that was that. Packaged foods were unheard of. All my friends grew up the same way, eating mostly fresh food with zero pre-packaged anything. And it seemed like we were consuming a *lot* of food. But what is even more astonishing, especially when I look back at the pictures or watch a movie from 50 years ago, is that no one was fat! I don't really remember a single person being overweight when I was young. Obesity, cancer, and heart disease were never mentioned."

"Oh my word, you are so right," Emily agreed. "Have you ever watched an old Annette Funicello movie with Frankie Avalon from the sixties? They were so lean! Everyone on TV was thin, as well as the rest of us! How do we get back to *that*?"

"It's very disconcerting how different it is now. The health of America is a staggering problem. Statistics tell us that money spent on the weight loss industry surpasses $20 billion per year![2] 108 million people are on diets in the United States on any given day. Dieters typically make 4 to 5 attempts per year.[3]

"So I echo your question, Emily. What in the world changed? And how can we get back there as soon as possible? What eating habits can we put back into our routine so we can live to see our great-great-grandkids grow up? How do we live a long, healthy life full of energy like they did back in the good 'old days?' "

"Yes," Emily agreed. "That's what I want to know. It seems so complicated now. I get emotional just thinking about food!"

"You're not alone, Emily. In all my years of personal-training, no other topic on the planet has produced as much confusion, disappointment, anger, shame, depression, and pain in people as the subject of food. It is a very emotionally-charged subject that can cause a lot of anxiety. To make matters worse, the nutrition rules keep changing. Our schedules are busier than ever which increases our propensity to grab fast food. And there are hundreds of diet plans that promise quick and easy results. No wonder the subject of food spans so many emotions and produces such exasperation in people."

"You know, Laurie, I didn't feel that way growing up. I never really thought about food except for when I was hungry. Now I think about it all the time and feel like it consumes a good part of my mental energy. And usually not in a good way. Most of my friends feel the same way—absolutely frustrated about what we should and shouldn't be eating. What in the world happened?"

"For starters, technology happened. Don't get me wrong, I love my computer, smart phone, iPad, and apps that help me do everything 100% faster than 10 years ago. The downside is that technology has morphed into how we play as well as work. We now sit more than any other generation."

"My chiropractor, Dr. David R. Mason, recently told me, 'Sitting has become the new smoking as far as unhealthy and detrimental risk factors. If I could only change one thing about everyone's lifestyle, it would be to sit as little as possible and move at every opportunity! I'd have a lot less business but people would see a new level of health and vitality. And that's a better way to live.' I couldn't agree with him more."

"Also, serving dishes are twice the size they were in the sixties. I remember shopping at a flea market recently with my daughter, Allie. We came across some vintage dinnerware that I recognized from my era. No doubt purchased with green stamps."

"Oh my goodness!" Emily recounted. "I remember those green stamps! That's a trip back in time. It seems like our dishes are enormous now compared to what they used to be. I remember dinnerware being *much* smaller back then."

"I know, right? As Allie held up a plate and marveled at the intricate detail she said, 'Oh, look, it's missing the dinner plates and just has these salad plates.' I had to laugh because I knew those small plates were the *dinner* plates! They were just so much smaller than what we're used to she thought they couldn't possibly be the right size. Talk about an object lesson right in front of us. Our dinner plates now are gigantic in comparison!

"I remember being interviewed on a local television station discussing America's obesity crisis. One of the issues I brought up was how plate sizes have dramatically increased in size. The host, Jennifer Hendricks, spoke right up and said, 'I know that to be true. I just bought a new set of dishes and they are too big for my standard-sized dishwasher!' While I appreciated the confirmation of her testimony, my heart sank a little too.

"From bagel shops to family restaurants to vending machines to movie theaters to the dining room table, meals and snacks are taking on gargantuan proportions. Marion Nestle, PhD, MPH, Professor of Nutrition and Food Studies at *New York University* stated 'Everyone in the food industry decided they had to make portions larger to stay competitive, and people got used to large sizes very quickly.'

"I couldn't agree with her more. Today normal sizes seem skimpy. The hyperinflation of our serving size is especially obvious away from home." Melanie Polk, registered dietitian and former director of nutrition education for the *American Institute of Cancer Research* said, 'Look through the window of any of the big chain restaurants, and you'll see huge dishes of food coming out of the kitchen. One of those large plates could easily pack 2,000 calories, enough to last most people all day. 25 years ago, the average American consumed about 1,850 calories each day. Since then, our daily consumption has grown by 304 calories—roughly the equivalent of 2 cans of soda. That's theoretically enough to add an extra 31 pounds to each person every year! Judging from the ongoing obesity epidemic, many Americans are suffering from those very consequences.⁴

Emily was flabbergasted. "31 pounds???? Holy guacamole!!"

"I know, Em! It's staggering, really. Because we live in a *super-size* culture and you can find a restaurant on practically every street corner, it makes competition for your dollars very high. Food is no longer served on plates—they use *platters!* And not the hey-everybody-dig-in kind of platter that feeds 4, but a single serving for *one* person! Restaurants are trying to provide the best bang for our buck so they're giving us bigger and bigger portions in hopes of winning our wallets.

"Portions are so predictably enormous now that my husband and I have gotten to a point where we almost always split a meal when eating out. I remember eating at an upscale restaurant a few years ago where we ordered a chicken breast meal to split. We usually start with salads so by the time the meal arrives *half* of the main entrée is the perfect size. But when our chicken arrived this time, the chef had already divided it onto two plates and each plate had two very large chicken breasts covering it. It was an impressive amount of food! I asked the waiter if he intentionally gave us more so my husband wouldn't starve! He's a big guy at 6 foot 5 inches and 210 pounds. The waiter responded, 'No, that's the usual portion size for this dish. The chef just split the regular amount onto two plates for your convenience.'"

"We couldn't believe our *half* portion was so immense! That half ended up being more than even my husband could finish and the total of both of our meals was *one* serving!"

"That's crazy, Laurie! I see it all the time too."

"Here's the thing, Emily. If we sit down to a serving like that and we're ravenous, there's a good chance we will eat most of it. Feeling overfull comes after the plate is empty. And that's a huge problem. Hunger can override "moderation" in a New York minute when the stomach is more than empty. The gut and the brain are always in communication but satiation is delayed by 15 to 20 minutes once we're full. I don't know about you, but if I'm super hungry I can consume a lot of food in those first 15 to 20 minutes! Then all of a sudden the brain gets the message from the gut that says, 'Hey, we're full down here. Shut off the appetite.' But by then we already feel stuffed. This has a profound effect on weight gain."

"I really think this has been a major influence in my struggle, Laurie."

"It's a common obstacle in our Standard American Diet that can keep us stuck and defeated. More than one-third—34.9% or 78.6 million—of U.S. adults are obese. Obesity-related conditions include heart disease, stroke, type 2 diabetes and certain types of cancer, which are some of the leading causes of preventable deaths. The estimated annual medical cost of obesity in the U.S. was $147 billion in 2008 U.S. dollars; the medical costs for people who are obese were $1,429 higher than those of normal weight.[5]

"Looking ahead, Emily, researchers have estimated that by 2030, if obesity trends continue unchecked, obesity-related medical costs alone could rise by $48 to $66 billion a year in the U.S."[6]

"Wow, that's alarming!"

"The two biggest problems with our health are that we move less, yet eat more. And the *more* of what we're eating isn't comprised enough of healthy farm-to-table vegetables and fruit, grass-fed organic meats, and free-range chickens like in the good old days. Too often it is from the prepackaged, grab-and-go aisle, void of any nutrition and loaded with sugar. That is not a sustainable way to live which is why America is in a health crisis."

"Good night, nurse! This is serious stuff. Show me the options you were talking about and let's get going on this thing!" Emily's motivation for change grew stronger every time we were together but I knew I needed to drive it home a little further.

"Before you can decide what you need to change, you need to assess where you are right now. Identify unhealthy traps you might fall into and discover any obstacles that might be influencing your health. I'll share with you the 5 most common and unhealthy patterns of eating that I personally succumbed to, which were also the same ones I observed while personally training thousands of clients over the years.

But let me lead off with the top 5 mistakes that permeated my own cycle of self-sabotage.

"If I were a betting person, I'd say one of those mistakes is sugar. It's got to be one of the top 5! I just know it. We all seem to struggle with this."

"Yep, you're right, Emily. **Mistake number 5 is too much sugar.** Gut health was relatively unheard of in the 80's, but now I understand that the bad bacteria in my gut was the root cause of my sugar cravings. I always just thought I had a sweet tooth that not everyone had. Now I understand that sugar keeps those little buggers alive and that's a big reason why craving sugar seems so hard to control. The bad bacteria in the gut is demanding them! And sugary temptations are everywhere! You can't even stop for gas without being bombarded with delectable donuts and hundreds of candy choices that never look better than when you've skipped a meal. So I constantly gave in! The more sugar I ate it, the more I needed! That was also a big reason I struggled to lose weight. The insulin released after eating sugar literally locks the door to a fat cell and makes us use sugar for energy instead of fat! It was a horrible addiction that kept me in bondage. And the sugar obsession in America seems to only be getting worse, and we rarely attribute it to the right cause: a gut that is unhealthy with bad bacteria overgrowth (Dysbiosis).

"It's very troubling, Emily. Despite our national obsession with weight loss, the obesity epidemic continues to be a national health hazard. With 170,000 fast-food restaurants and 3 million soft-drink vending machines spread across the country, huge doses of sugar calories are never far away—especially when those soda machines are sitting right in the middle of public schools. In 1978 the typical teen-age boy in the United States drank about 7 ounces of soda a day, according to *Fast Food Nation* author Eric Schlosser. Today, the typical teen-age boy drinks nearly three times that much, getting a whopping 9% of his daily calories from soda! Teenage girls are close behind."[6]

"Oh, my goodness," Emily interjected, "170,000 fast food choices?? That boggles the mind and is just downright scary to think about for our kids."

"You're right, Emily. It's not good in any way, shape, or form. We're now starting to discover that sugar is a major player in heart disease. *The Saint Luke's Mid America Heart Institute* and *Albert Einstein College of Medicine* research states that they are finding a higher incidence of heart disease. They are concerned that consuming large quantities of sugar such as high fructose corn syrup and table sugar, can lead to leptin resistance—leptin, remember, is a hormone responsible for shutting off appetite and regulating normal body weight. Foods high in sugars also promote type 2 diabetes which can lead to a much greater risk for coronary heart disease.[7] The researchers were interested in seeing what's worse for the heart—saturated fats or refined sugars. Their findings published in *Progress in Cardiovascular Diseases* argue that, after years of believing fat was worse, more than likely *sugar* is the major culprit."

"Why is sugar so bad if it has half the calories of fat?" Emily asked.

"When you eat something with sugar in it, even if it is fruit, your body releases insulin to regulate your blood sugar. Over time this can cause your blood cells to become insulin resistant, meaning the insulin is no longer effective in regulating your blood sugar. This is known as pre-diabetes and is a precursor to developing Type 2 diabetes which is a leading driver of many diseases including metabolic syndrome, obesity, and cardiovascular disease."[8]

"Oh, for the love of Pete! All the sugar I've consumed over the years!"

"Emily, I'm right there with you. My husband had a health scare just last year. He's normally very active, plays racquetball twice a week and runs half marathons! He kept complaining of shortness of breath, an erratic heart rate, and major fatigue and finally had some blood work done. The doc called him at home to tell him his lab results showed blood sugar issues! Fortunately we learned about gut health, eliminated sugar from our foods as much as possible, and started him on some natural, plant-based supplements and probiotics. Within one month all his symptoms went away! He wanted proof that he wasn't just imagining he was better so he had his doc run all his labs again and the numbers were normal!"

"That's fantastic, Laurie! I want to know more about how he did that!"

"We'll chat about that later but first let's finish with my other 4 mistakes. That way you can learn the easy way and avoid the same pitfalls that kept me exhausted and unable to lose weight.

"Well, number five was a doozy, that's for sure!"

"They will all have an impact on how you look, feel, and live. The fourth biggest mistake also contributed to my poor gut health and that was eating **too many trans-fats**."

"This is not to be confused with the good fats we get from nuts and lean meat. Trans-fats are considered by most nutritional professionals to be the worst type of fat you can eat. Unlike other dietary fats, trans-fats—also called trans-fatty acids—both raise your LDL (*bad*) cholesterol and lower your HDL (*good*) cholesterol. A high LDL level in combination with a low HDL level increases your risk of heart disease, the leading killer of men and women, as you know.[9] Most trans-fat is formed through an industrial process that adds hydrogen to vegetable oil which causes the oil to become solid at room temperature. Picture something like lard or mayonnaise. But it can be found lurking in many foods."

"Yeah, that's what I thought. Darn it."

"This partially hydrogenated oil is less likely to spoil so foods made with it have a longer shelf life. Some restaurants use partially hydrogenated vegetable oil in their deep fryers since it doesn't have to be changed as often as do other oils."

"There's a reason. It's cheaper, right?" Emily asked.

"Exactly," I responded. "But it's not just limited to lard and mayonnaise. It's in tons of other foods that are processed."

"Like what?" Emily probed. "Can I have a list? I work better with lists in front of me and you seem to have one in your back pocket at all times," Emily teased.

"As a matter of fact," I said laughing, "I can give you a list right now."

"See? That's what I'm talkin' about. Fire away, please."

"Keep in mind that these are the usual culprits unless they are specifically labeled that they do not have trans-fat in them. Some manufacturers are trying to find healthier ways to produce their products without trans-fat since it has gotten huge negative publicity in the past few years. Although there are many others, the big offenders are baked goods like donuts, cookies, cakes, and brownies, canned frostings, coffee creamer, margarine, snacks like crackers, bars, and chips. Potato, corn and tortilla chips often contain trans-fat unless listed on the label. And while popcorn *can* be a healthy snack if you make it at home with coconut oil and real popping corn, many types of packaged or microwave popcorn use trans-fat to help cook or flavor the popcorn."

"Also, foods that require deep frying—French fries, tortilla chips, and fried chicken—can contain trans-fat from the oil used in the cooking process. Another big player is refrigerated dough such as canned biscuits, cinnamon rolls, and frozen pizza crusts often contain trans-fat."[10]

"Well, for Pete's sake, is there any food left to eat?" Emily asked sarcastically.

"Oh, and another important reason to avoid processed foods is because they're high in MSG (Monosodium Glutamate), which is linked to symptoms such as headaches, allergies, inflammation, and brain fog. MSG has also been blamed for *increasing* hunger since you can eat a ton of it and it never registers satiation to the brain because *it's not real food*. It's enhanced chemicals and additives that have been manufactured by companies to resemble food and taste appealing. Ever been starving and reached for a bag of cheese puffs?"

"Me? No. I would never do that." Emily teased.

"Well, unfortunately I know by experience that you can eat half the bag and still be hungry because it's void of any healthy nutrients. Add in the sweeteners, colors, dyes, artificial flavors, and nitrites that are often added to processed foods and you've got quite a chemical cocktail. There's a reason it's called junk food—it's junk, not food!"

"Ouch. Harsh, but true."

"As I shared with you, I used to really struggle here. I was at a very dark time in my life and turned to food—and I use the term *food* loosely. I used it for comfort, not nutrition. Food was always there with no condemnation. Until I realized that NONE of my clothes fit me anymore! 35 pounds later, I began to notice my *comfort foods* were not in the least bit comforting. They were producing major anxiety! And now I know that all of these trans-fats were wreaking havoc on my gut health—an extra whammy!

"You've earned your stripes, Laurie. There's nothing more helpful than someone who has walked in your shoes and knows firsthand how hard it is to change. You understand from the depths of your toes. You've struggled. You've probably even suffered it sounds like. So you can bet I'm listening and taking all of this to heart."

"That's why I share all this, Em. I don't want you to make the same mistakes I did. Like the next one—number 3 was **not eating foods high in fiber.**"

"I already know I'm not getting enough of this," Emily confessed.

"Turns out we need a lot of fiber, Emily! We need 25-30 grams of fiber but most people only get 12-15 grams, less than half of what is recommended. I know I was probably way below even 12 grams since I rarely ate vegetables—and definitely *not* nuts. I mistakenly thought the fat in nuts made me fat," I admitted.

"So here's what we know about fiber. Fiber is commonly classified as *soluble*, which dissolves in water, or *insoluble*, which doesn't dissolve." I explained, "Soluble fiber dissolves in water to form a gel-like material. It can help lower blood cholesterol and glucose levels. Soluble fiber can be found in foods like oats, peas, beans, apples, citrus fruits, carrots, barley and psyllium.

"And then there is insoluble fiber. This type of fiber promotes the movement of material through your digestive system and increases stool bulk. This helps prevent conditions like diverticular disease and constipation so it is of great benefit."[12]

"This is another one for Jeffrey," Emily whispered.

"Insoluble fiber can be found in wheat bran, nuts, beans and vegetables. Foods like cauliflower, green beans, potatoes, brown rice, legumes, carrots, cucumbers and tomatoes are a great source of insoluble fiber. Most plant-based foods such as beans and oatmeal contain *both* soluble and insoluble fiber. However, the amount of each type varies in different plant foods so it works best to eat a wide variety of high-fiber foods.

"One of the greatest benefits of high-fiber foods is that they tend to be more filling than low-fiber foods. So you're likely to eat less and stay satisfied longer. Once I understood how much I needed fiber and started consuming a lot more veggies, I could stay fuller longer. That meant I ate less food but was never starving."

"Now I like that—no starving."

"Absolutely no starving ever again," I reassured her.

Emily nodded her head in agreement, took a deep breath, and sighed in relief.

"Emily, it this way: If God made it, eat it. If man made it, don't eat it. That means the foods God made are real. Man-made foods have been stripped of their natural nutrients and that often means fiber. The grain-refining process removes the outer coat (bran) from the grain, which lowers its fiber content. Enriched foods have some of the B vitamins and iron back after processing, but not the fiber."[13]

"Good to know. Eat real food that God made. Does that mean I can have potatoes?"

"Did God make them?"

"He sure did."

"Then I say yes. They have a little bit more sugar so just use moderation with them but they are loaded with nutrients, especially sweet potatoes. Get your fiber from plants and add digestive enzymes from your plant-based supplements."

Okay, lots of helpful info here. I'm stoked about having potatoes back in my life—in moderation. Loving it."

"Great, Em. Let's move on to my **second biggest mistake which was skipping breakfast.** I thought by skipping breakfast I was saving calories. But food is—above all things—fuel. People who skip breakfast are not giving their bodies an opportunity to *break-fast.* Your body has been without fuel, *fasting,* if you will, for 10 to 12 hours depending on when you eat dinner and when you wake. Regardless of the exact timing, that is a long time to go without fuel. Breakfast is the perfect time to prepare the engine for the day ahead, stoking it at regular intervals for peak energy.

"Researchers at the *Harvard School of Public Health* recently did a study on older men who skipped breakfast and what they found was alarming. Those who regularly skipped breakfast had a 27% higher risk of a heart attack than those who ate a morning meal! There's no reason why the results wouldn't apply to people of all ages too, the *Harvard* researchers said.[6]

"Why would skipping breakfast increase a heart attack risk?" Emily asked.

"Experts aren't certain but here's what they think: People who don't eat breakfast are more likely to be hungrier later in the day and eat larger meals. Those bigger meals mean that the body must process a larger amount of calories in a shorter amount of time. That can spike sugar levels in the blood and perhaps even lead to clogged arteries."

"But is a stack of syrupy pancakes, greasy eggs and lots of bacon really better than eating nothing?"

"Other experts agreed that it's hard to say." I replied. "Andrew Odegaard, a *University of Minnesota* researcher who has studied a link between skipping breakfast and health problems like obesity and high blood pressure said, 'We don't know whether it's the timing or content of breakfast that's important. It's probably both. Generally, people who eat breakfast tend to eat healthier through the day.'"[14]

"So basically your brain thinks if you skip breakfast, you're starving. So it ramps up your appetite at night to make up for the missed breakfast." Emily summarized succinctly.

"Yes, that seems to be the case," I replied.

"What if you're not a breakfast eater at all? Should you force yourself to eat?

"Eat breakfast when it's reasonable for you. If you get up at 6 AM but don't really feel hungry until 9 AM, eat then," I answered.

"That's a reasonable plan."

"This leads us to the number one mistake. Drum roll please."

"The suspense is killing me," Emily said, trying to hurry me.

"Emily, **dieting is the number one mistake to avoid at *all* costs!**"

"Well it's about flippin' time somebody said diets don't work! I feel like I've been on a diet my whole life and where has it gotten me—besides cranky?"

"You don't ever have to *diet* again, Emily. But just to make sure you're never tempted by it again, let's talk about *why* diets don't work."

I explained, "Dieting is a temporary fix. We all know people who have gone on *diets* and lost weight. Yes, most people can lose weight! But about 95% of the people that lose weight on a diet will gain it back within 3 years, according to Gary D. Foster, PhD, Director, *Center for Obesity Research and Education*, Professor of Medicine and Public Health.[2] Since dieting by definition is a temporary food restriction, it won't work in the long run. Moreover, the deprivation of restrictive diets may lead to a diet-overeat or diet-binge cycle, which is exactly what happened to me. And since your body doesn't want you to starve, it responds to overly-restrictive diets by slowing your metabolism which of course makes it harder to lose weight even though you're eating next to nothing."

"Fad diets can be incredibly harmful. They usually lack basic essential nutrients and some even warn users *not* to use the diet long term! That should be a red flag right there. For 6 weeks you power through and eat in a way that is not sustainable but you're not learning to eat *better*, you're just eating *less*. Thus, when you've *completed* your fad diet timeframe you simply boomerang back to the unhealthy eating patterns that caused your weight gain in the first place! This is known as *yo-yo dieting*, which is very traumatic to your body, your heart health, and your emotions!"

"It's an awful way to live and I've had just about enough of it."

"I agree, Em. It works against us in so many ways. Dieting can also lead to eating disorders. According to Alice Covey, RD CD, dieting may not be the cause of *all* eating disorders, but it is often a powerful precursor. *The National Eating Disorders Association* reports that 35% of *normal dieters* progress to pathological dieting, and that 20-25% of those individuals develop eating disorders. It is far too common that eating disorders start off as dieting.[15]

I explained, "So the first step towards permanent healthy weight loss is, somewhat ironically, to **lose the diet** and the diet mindset. Instead, think about food as fuel that you can enjoy for the rest of your life. How boring! How prosaic! Yet how true."[16]

I confessed, once again, the heartbreak—and wisdom—I had gained from my own terrible experiences. "You know, Emily, in the past I made every nutritional mistake in the book. I let it run my life. The truth is God created food for us to enjoy and never intended for it to make us feel guilty, ashamed, or confused. It's meant to provide the sustenance we need so we can get on with the things that matter most—loving well, serving others, living out our calling, and stepping into our dreams for the future. Food should be a complement to all of *that*, not the center of it."

"Oh how true. I've got a lot of living—and loving—to do, and I'm so tired of food getting in the way of my health, energy, and peace. It's been the focus for far too long. It should be helping me, not hurting me," Emily said with resolve.

"You're ready for that, Emily. I've seen a new level of courage rising up in you. As you've been transforming your mind and heart, and adding the new tools of water, sleep, exercise and now clean eating, you are becoming a new person. You're developing the mindset of a warrior—determined, fearless, and unrelenting. I'm so proud of the steps you've taken to change who you are as a person, attempting new challenges that before seemed daunting and impossible. With all those new tools in your arsenal, food is the final frontier. It's just one more battle you're going to win to live an extraordinary life. "

"Honestly, I could have never accomplished any of this on my own. I feel like for the first time in my life that I am headed in a whole new direction and none of it is complicated, gimmicky, or difficult. I already feel so much better. I have new energy and peace in my life. I'm praying all the time, not just at night. Who would've ever guessed that!

"But most importantly, Laurie, I have…" Emily struggled as she searched for the right words, "…I have a beautiful thing called *hope*."

"From the beginning, this process has sharpened and refined me as a person. I know I've been a tough nut to crack but you didn't give up. I'm not the same guilt-ridden, shackled-by-shame, afraid-of-the-smallest-change Emily anymore. My mind and heart are apprehending the challenges you place in front of me with courage and determination. For the first time in forever, I am really starting to feel fearless. And that has been the best part of this journey."

"Emily, we'll have our last session tomorrow so I'm giving you some homework tonight called "I AM." I want you to dig deep and make a list of all that you've become and all that you still want to be. Take a blank piece of paper and write I AM at the top. Then fill in who you've become in one line sentences with as many as you can think of. You are strong. You are disciplined. You are incredible! When you say the words "I am" you are speaking the identity God gave you. What does He say about you? That's your assignment for tonight. Write who God says you are with authority and promise."

This will become your new script that you say to yourself every single day. And you know what? The more you say it, the more you will believe it and *that* will change your life too! One thing I daily say to myself is that "I AM free from shame!" For so much of my life, shame was a label—an identity—that I took into my heart and soul every time I made a mistake or failed at something. It kept me paralyzed from taking chances and trying new things, but mostly it stopped me from chasing my dreams and believing that I could be who God had designed me to be. Now every morning this is what I say:

I AM who God says I am:
A light-bearer
A hope bringer
A courage giver
A joy lifter

I AM a warrior:
Strong and courageous
Mighty in all my work
Fierce against opposition
Surrounded by your songs of victory
Positioned for miraculous success

I AM a writer:
Carefully listening to the language of your Holy Spirit
Boldly announcing your message of love to the world
Fearlessly sharing the truth you place on my heart and mind

I AM a dearly loved child:
Made in your image
Covered by the blood of Jesus, completely forgiven
With full authority over all things and situations

When I say 'I AM' I really believe it and I set my day on that very powerful truth."

"Oh, Laurie, I've been so riddled with guilt and shame from food, from my weight, from my inability to control my emotions, my anger, food....there's a long list really. And all of it has stolen my ability to believe in myself, my dreams, and my calling. I will definitely do this assignment tonight and make sure I include all the parts of me that are new and all the beautiful future parts I hope to yet become. Here's one for you—I AM HOPEFUL! You like that one? Never mind, I already know you do," Emily laughed.

Oh Em…it's one of my favorites. It's the opposite of shame and it will light your path so you can find brand new things inside of you. Hope. It's a small word. But miraculous to every person it touches.

Chapter 8
Fuel Your Body...For Real...With REAL Food

"Hope fans the flame of transformation and that is the warrior strength you're seeing within yourself."

I'll never forget the kind women who spoke life and courage over me 3 decades ago. Before they ever saw a kernel of that truth being lived out in me, they believed they would. Their words still resonate in my soul today. When I was struggling to even lift my chin, their love and prophetic words were a healing balm to my aching spirit as they helped me believe magnificent days were ahead. They treated me like the person I could become, not the one I was or had been. And that was the same language of love that was now flowing over Emily.

The next morning as Emily and I met for the last time, I poured out as much encouragement as possible. "All the changes you've made so far have dramatically increased your energy and strength physically, spiritually, and emotionally. Your determination is inspiring! You've been willing to make some very tough decisions and have applied all the tools you've learned with tenacity and commitment. The amazing progress you see has been created from your own resolve and discipline."

Emily's eyes lit up. "I'm not going to be deterred this time. I do feel stronger! A *lot* stronger. These tools are simple and yet they are really making a difference in how I feel. I gotta hand it to you."

"And I'm handing it right back to you! It's been *you* making the changes, not me. I can only offer information and recommendations. What you do when you walk out these doors is completely up to you. *You* decide when and how much water to drink. *You* decide what habits to use through the day to help you sleep better. *You* decide how to move and play and exercise and *you* decide what clean food to eat. It's you, baby, all the way."

Emily smiled, acknowledging all the work she had done. "I don't feel like the same me that started this program. There's a deeper hunger to stay consistent with these tools and a growing confidence that I can and will not give up! I see myself making headway every day and that is beyond exciting."

"That's awesome, Em."

"I still want to know how you lost weight without going on a diet," she prodded, not letting me off the hook.

"As it turns out, that's our focus for today."

"Oh, good," Emily said, excitedly. "Finally! I've been waiting for this one."

"After trying all the ridiculous and shame-producing *diets* 30 years ago, I was finally able to lose 35 pounds and keep it off by following a simple plan of eating REAL food and getting my gut healthy so my body could work for me, not against me. My food choices brought healing instead of anxiety, and that changed everything.

"When friends saw that I was losing weight—and keeping it off—they wanted to know the *secret*. And by "secret" they wanted to know which diet I was using. Well, here's the secret: I learned how to *eat real food*, not how to diet! Food deprivation through dieting *doesn't work!* It lowers our quality of life and is oppressive to our spirits. As a matter of fact, dieting actually helps us gain weight because it lowers our metabolism!

"I love what actress Totie Fields once said: 'I've been a diet for 2 weeks and all I've lost is 14 days!'"

"That sounds about right," Emily agreed, laughing.

"Emily, you've been very successful with planning the other three tools involving water, sleep, and exercise. You did that because your health, energy, and peace are very important to you. We plan the things that are a priority. We just do. So let's keep that same mindset and plan what we eat."

"Absolutely! I'm determined to conquer this food thing, ramp up my energy, and lose weight the right way. Forever! And then there's that whole mountain thing."

"Fantastic, Em! There's so much to celebrate and plan for. Let me provide 7 practical ideas to help you choose real foods that are delicious and fabulously good for you all at the same time. These recommendations are compiled from what I used years ago to get on track and what I use now to stay on track. Losing weight is simply a by-product of using what's in your toolbox, moment by moment, day by day, week by week. We know that clean eating has a massive impact on our gut health and that helps our bodies work for us in a powerful way to maintain a healthy weight. The way we eat should never be something we go on and off of. It needs to be a sustainable plan for the rest of our lives.

"Amen to that!" Emily exclaimed, approvingly.

"It's also important to abide by the Glycemic Index which is a nutritional measure of how carbohydrates affect our levels of blood sugar. While I didn't know about the Glycemic Index 30 years ago, it is a very effective way to gauge which carbs are lower in sugar. The higher the Glycemic Index number, the faster our blood sugar levels rise. That releases insulin in our body. And insulin makes us *store* fat. The lower the number on the Glycemic Index, the slower the carbohydrate makes our blood sugar rise which is definitely what we want. Stick to the foods that don't get your blood sugar out of whack. It doesn't matter if you're diabetic or not, sustained blood sugar should be a goal for everyone. High blood sugar can cause weight gain, headaches, heart disease, and increase your risk of type 2 diabetes.

"I have such bad sugar cravings. Is there anything that can help that? I feel completely powerless, even when I have the strongest intentions. It makes me feel so weak." Emily confessed, reluctantly.

"You know, Emily. I have battled sugar cravings my entire life. I started to think it was in my DNA! I had no idea my gut health was the culprit. There are bad bacteria and good bacteria that live together in your gut, and you always want to proportionally have more good to avoid dysbiosis, an unhealthy ratio where the bad bacteria outnumber the good. Once I started to learn about my gut environment and that the bad bacteria and Candida overgrowth actually *live on sugar*, I started to understand how to fight it. The more prolific the good bacteria becomes, the less bad bacteria can thrive. Gut health supplements helped me kill the bad guys and grow the good guys."

"Oh my goodness! Boooooo! Death to the bad bacteria!" Emily exclaimed. "I've heard about gut health but I really don't understand all the details. It actually makes me mad that the bad bacteria and Candida overgrowth are making me crave sugar *for them!* Talk about free rent! They are powerful little guys, aren't they? How can I get more good ones in my gut?"

"Clean eating is essential, Emily. Eat real food all the time. Every day. Every meal. And don't forget to eat probiotics. Foods that are rich in good bacteria like Greek yogurt, Kefir, Sauerkraut, fermented cheeses, and Kombucha are natural probiotics."

"Kom-who-a?" Emily teased.

"Kombucha. I know the names are a little weird but they are full of good guys!"

"Doesn't "good bacteria" sound like an oxymoron? And you're saying I need more of them?"

"Yes, Em. It's imperative that you have enormous amounts of good bacteria and decrease bad bacteria. Too many of the bad guys and you can experience a "leaky gut" which can lead to many horrible health issues. Your gut is also responsible for 70% of your immune health and 90% of your brain hormones like serotonin, dopamine, and melatonin."

"Ah, yes. I remember chatting about melatonin during our sleep session. So if my gut helps makes melatonin, are you saying a healthy gut will help me sleep better?" Emily surmised.

"Yes, ma'am. It has an immense effect. Your gut has over 100 trillion microbes and health experts call it our "second brain.""

"How cool is that! So probiotics help increase my good bacteria, but how do I get rid of the bad bacteria? And will that help me lose weight?"

"Bad bacteria have a hard shell protecting them called Chitin and they can actually burrow into your intestinal walls and cause holes called Leaky Gut. Your intestinal walls can leak your nutrients from food and your waste into your bloodstream! That makes inflammation proliferate throughout your body which can me you very sick. The supplements I use actually dissolve that hard shell and kill the bad bacteria. I've done a ton of research on the ingredients and I have to say they have all made such a difference in how I feel. The sugar cravings I've had all my life were extremely stubborn, but now they're gone completely. Also when you heal your Leaky Gut, you can help heal the rest of your body."

"Holy cow, Laurie! I need to add this to my routine! I know if it works for you, it will work for me and I love that the supplements are made from plants. With gut health making the news so often I don't want to overlook this."

"Emily, I gave birth without medication—that's how paranoid I am about what goes into my body. So taking all natural supplements made from organic plants was very important to me. It just made sense to us that God would use his creation—his plants—to help his kids feel better."

"Yep, it sure does."

"Just remember that vitamins and supplements are tools, like water, sleep, exercise, and clean eating. They're not a cure-all and none of them alone can give us optimal health."

"I'm sure learning that!" Emily declared. "I always thought I just needed a good diet for about 10 weeks so I could lose 20 pounds. Now I see that while the tools themselves are simple, the process inside your body and mind is a lot more complicated. So many factors enter into our journey towards better health. But now I know that a good "diet" doesn't exist."

"Wow, listen to you! You'll be taking over for me in no time!"

"No, no. I'll leave all the training up to you. But I do want to hear more about clean eating and how to fit that into my daily routine."

I handed Emily a printout of her final tool. A sustainable eating plan based on "clean" foods. I began to explain, "So here's my Golden 7 Plan that I used to get healthy and lose weight. These 7 principles made it easier to kick my old habits to the curb and implement the ones that could save me from my bad choices. Through this, I learned to appreciate my meals instead of feeling ashamed every time I ate."

"Well let's get to it!" Emily prodded.

"**Number 1: say a prayer of thanks every time you eat.** Once I started to be grateful for the food going in my belly instead of feeling guilty, I lost the anxiety I had at every mealtime. Food is a gift. And millions of people don't have that gift each day. Let's not take it for granted. The United Nations Food and Agriculture Organization estimates that about 795 million of the 7.3 billion people in the world, or 1 person in 9, suffered from chronic undernourishment in 2014-2016.[1]"

"That's a staggering number! I'm not going to let food shame me anymore. It really is a *gift*! Saying a prayer of thanks is a great first step."

"**Number 2: Lose the junk.** I emptied my house of all sugar, artificial sweeteners, and white flour foods! Nothing says *I'm committed* like clearing out the pantry and fridge of all processed and packaged foods. Don't tempt yourself with foods that don't help you become stronger or make you feel better. Make a commitment to use only "clean" foods that are one ingredient—the ones that God made—and watch your food become your medicine.

"**Number 3: Add complex carbs through plants.** Once I started eating more complex carbs, which went against what every *diet* told me to do, I got a new level of energy and started feeling remarkably better."

I explained what changes I made, "I chose a meal plan that was high in complex carbs, mostly veggies, a little fruit, and a smidge of grains like oats and barley."

"So carbs are good?" Emily asked.

"Yep. Of course I'm talking about the plant kind of carbohydrates. The cookies, crackers, breads, and donut types that are processed and refined literally made my gut sick, which made my whole body inflamed. Complex carbohydrates keep us supplied with energy, fiber, and nutrients that only plants can provide. Your carbs should be mostly vegetables, all organic. This comprises about 33% or 1/3 of all your foods in a day. And of course, always a good idea to add protein and fats at the same time.

"There are many, many benefits of plant-based carbs. Foods from plant sources fight inflammation which has been linked to many diseases like cancer, heart disease, diabetes, and arthritis. The fiber in plants will keep your digestive systems working properly, provide satiation to your appetite, help keep blood sugar balanced, and keep you feeling fuller so you don't overeat. This also makes it easier to lose weight."

Emily smiled, "We're on the right track here. You have my undivided attention."

"Next," I explained, "I ate spinach or kale salads almost nightly and munched on colorful veggies which helped me fill up on rich nutrients so I didn't need second helpings of the main dish. This is still a habit I use today. A salad with lunch or dinner is a great way to pile on the produce and prevent overconsumption of large main entrees. Just make sure the dressing is clear, not creamy, and is preferably some type of organic balsamic with EVOO (Extra Virgin Olive Oil). I've got a wonderful balsamic recipe for you to try. I also added plenty of nuts, seeds, and avocados for good fat which makes a salad satiating."

I talked more about vegetable choices, "I chose vegetables that were dark and rich in color. Among the top vegetable choices are spinach, bell peppers, cucumbers, green beans, and kale. Anything dark and leafy always makes a good choice, as well as, cruciferous vegetables like cauliflower, broccoli, collard greens, and cabbage. These are non-starchy vegetables that pack a punch against disease and can be easily eaten without cooking.

"Starchy vegetables generally are not as easy to eat in their raw form since they are roots, bulbs, or kernels. These starchy vegetables include sweet potatoes, squash, corn, peas, pumpkin, zucchini, beets, and carrots. They also rate higher on the glycemic index, so eat more non-starchy veggies for sugar balance but know they are both loaded with vitamins and antioxidants. An excellent first choice to any meal."

"Any meal? Even breakfast?"

"Sure. Think veggie omelet. Throw leftover veggies from dinner into a pan with avacado or coconut oil and whip them into some eggs. Or keep them chopped up for easy access at every meal, including breakfast. Once I ate my veggies first I felt so much better at the end of a meal because I didn't overeat. Sound doable, Em?"

"Yep. Throwing veggies in an omelet is a simple, easy, and realistic plan for me to prepare breakfast in the mornings. This will be a cinch."

"Fruit, used sparingly because of its sugar content, became my dessert. The best way to keep insulin from being released when eating fruit is to combine it with a good fat. Try using almond butter. Or throw a few sliced almonds or walnuts on top of yogurt with a berry combo.

"Here's what I do almost every night now: I add 2 cups of spinach, 2 tablespoons of milled flax seed and chia seeds, 1 tablespoon of organic coconut oil or coconut kefir, 1 tablespoon of almond butter or a scoop of Plexus chocolate protein called Lean, a few blueberries, fill it up with water or almond milk, add the lid to the top, and stick it in the fridge. Then in the morning, I blend it for about 10 seconds and voila!"

"2 cups of spinach?" Emily groaned.

"Trust me, you don't even taste the spinach with a little bit of fruit in there. It's rich in antioxidants and polyphenols, completely satiating, and oh-so-delish. Play with the flavor. Make it your own and create a special blend that you love. I recently started adding a little Acai to it which is delish."

I had to confess, "Before I got my gut healthy and was addicted to sugar, I forgot how sweet ripe fruit tasted. I often refer to it as *God's candy*. In the smoothie, I added organic dark-colored fruit like blackberries, blueberries, cherries, and raspberries, which are all wonderful and full of healing properties.

"Like vegetables, there are really no bad choices of fruit. The juicier fruits like watermelons, oranges and grapefruits are great for hydration since they contain a lot of water. Fruits contain important phytonutrients and antioxidants that boost our immune systems, improve how well our body metabolizes food, help prevent disease, and protect our health."

With a knowing wink I mentioned Emily's favorite food. "Other food modifications for me involved limiting bread. I stopped eating anything with white flour which helped me feel less bloated, gassy and achy. I significantly reduced grains. Most bread is completely over-processed and full of gluten, a known cause of inflammation. Healthier grain choices are oats (make sure they are certified organic and gluten-free since oats can easily be cross-contaminated in the processing plants that refine wheat), quinoa, spelt, or buckwheat. There are some wonderful gluten-free options now in just about every food category substituting for white flour. If you do have whole wheat bread, make sure there are no artificial ingredients or sugar added and the grain should be as unprocessed as possible."

I went on to discuss other foods that may give the impression from the label that they are healthy, but in fact are not, "**Number 4: Add good fats and stop eating low-fat**. I stopped eating *fat-free* and fake *low-fat* foods when I learned the value of healthy fats and added nuts, seeds, healthy meats, and coconut and olive oil to my diet. This helped me stay fuller longer and lose more weight. We *need* good fats. Seriously! Fats don't make us fat."

Emily interjected, "Okay, can we stop right here for a sec? I'm having a hard time with this one. I'm working so hard to get healthy and lose weight. I don't want to blow it. Don't fats have more calories than carbs or proteins?"

"The short answer is yes, Emily. But they do a ton of good things for you so you need them in your plan. I haven't led you astray so far, have I?" I asked.

"No. No, you haven't. I trust you. I'm just not used to saying "good" in front of fats," Emily admitted.

"It's okay. Maybe it will make more sense once I explain exactly what they do"

"That might help," Emily answered.

"I used to be scared to death of fats way back when I was struggling with my weight. Here's the truth. We need plenty of monounsaturated and polyunsaturated fats. They are essential components of cell membranes. They help with nutrient absorption, nerve transmission, and maintaining cell membrane integrity. They also help provide energy during sustained exercise and in between meals. In addition to all of those jobs, they also insulate and act as a shock absorber for bones and organs."[2]

I continued, "They also help lower the risk of heart disease and stroke by lowering triglyceride and cholesterol levels and reducing plaque buildup in the arteries.[3] They're powerful anti-inflammatories that have the added bonus of contributing incredible flavor to food and providing delicious satiation!

"Some of my top choices for monounsaturated fats are avocadoes, olives, nuts like almonds, macadamias, pecans, cashews, and natural almond butter. For polyunsaturated fats which are higher in Omega-3's, I like flaxseed (make sure it's milled), walnuts, pumpkin seeds, and wild fatty fish like trout or salmon."

"What about the fats I cook with?"

"When you choose fats in the form of oils make sure that the olive oil is EVOO which is the highest quality and most expensive olive oil classification. EVOO must be produced entirely by mechanical means, without the use of any solvents, by cold-pressing and using temperatures that will not degrade the oil. EVOO is somewhat fragile and appropriate for low to medium cooking, not high heat which breaks down its components."

Emily asked, "EVOO is the most expensive?"

I answered, "Yes. But it's one of those nutrient-dense choices that is well worth a couple more dollars."

Emily agreed, so I continued, "Coconut, avocado, and ghee are good oils to cook with for high heat and can be refined. The bottom line is that fats in the form of monounsaturated and polyunsaturated are super healthy for us and keep us full longer, which is also incredibly helpful in losing weight. Even a fat like butter, even though saturated, can be consumed since it is *real* food. Fats should comprise 1/3 of what we eat."

"That seems like a big percentage—33%?"

"That's correct, Emily. Remember, good fats are *good*. Especially those high in Omega-3 fatty acids."

"Complex carb—1/3 of all we eat. Fats—1/3. That still leaves 1/3 left. Wine and dessert?" Emily joked.

"The final 33% is **Number 5: Add good proteins**. This is what helped my hair stop falling out 35 years ago. There are many options for protein intake. It doesn't mean just meat.

"It seems like there is so much controversy over meat these days. Strict vegetarians don't ever eat meat. I have several friends that are vegetarians and also vegans (no dairy), and they are healthy and happy. I also have friends that are strictly paleo. Equally happy and healthy."

"Honestly I don't think I get enough protein. I have mistakenly put it in the same category as fat that makes me fat, afraid it was not the healthiest choice."

"I can tell you what worked for me—and hundreds of my clients—when protein took its rightful place in the eating plan. First of all, protein is an important component of every cell in the body and is a building block for bones, muscles, cartilage, skin, and blood. Hair and nails are mostly made of protein. Your body uses protein to build and repair tissues, to make enzymes, hormones, and other chemicals in the body.

"Along with fat and carbohydrates, protein is a *macronutrient*, meaning that the body needs relatively large amounts of it. Vitamins and minerals, which are needed in only small quantities, are called *micronutrients*. But unlike fat and carbohydrates, the body does not store protein and therefore has no reservoir to draw on when it needs a new supply."[5]

I emphasized, "We need protein to balance out our health and nutrition, and fortunately there are a lot of options to include it. Protein from animal sources should be as close to natural as possible.

It's fairly easy today to find local farmers at farmer's markets where you can buy a variety of meats directly. Ask them about their practices. Some may be certified organic, which means that the *USDA* has certified that animals grazed certified organic lands. The animals must be organic fed and cannot be treated with growth hormones or antibiotics since that's passed to you when you eat it. Antibiotics kill our good bacteria so make sure all your meat is organic.

"Mike and I buy directly from organic farmers whenever possible and it's amazing how much better the meat tastes. It's also more abundant in grocery stores under the organic label, but you can't beat fresh from the farmer. Or fresh fish from the ocean that just melts in your mouth."

"Another source of protein is eggs. Over time eggs have been in vogue and then out and then back in."

"I know. Would they please make up their minds?"

"Eggs are a very good source of protein for you, Emily, since you're not a vegan. Again, if you can find them directly from a local farmer you're likely to get eggs that are high in omega-3 fat containing DHA. That's good brain food. Eggs also contain choline, lutein for our eye health, and B vitamins essential for our health."

"Other great options for protein are nuts, seeds, beans, and hummus. One of my favorite *super-foods* is hummus. I always keep hummus stocked in my fridge and I've also included a tasty homemade recipe for you. It's made from garbanzo beans, also commonly known as chickpeas, which are rich in protein and carbohydrates, along with olive oil (good fat), Tahini, a sesame paste containing good fats and protein, garlic, lemon, and herbs. Hummus is a tasty, healthy, fantastic, meatless source of protein also high in omega-3 fats."

"Oh, I love hummus," Emily responded. "And now that I know it's a *super-food*, I love it even more."

"It really will make a difference in your health when you start adding the right amount of protein to your eating plan."

"Wow, I can definitely make some better choices here," Emily offered. "And, by the way, your hair looks lovely."

"It's amazing what clean foods in the right amounts can do for your entire body including your hair and nails! No more clumps falling out for this girl!"

"Yes more protein it is!"

"Number 6: Start the day with breakfast. Not a bowl of fruit loops. Not a bagel on the way out the door. When I started the day with a nutrient-packed breakfast instead of skipping it to save calories or jamming a sugar fix down my throat, I noticed I wasn't ravenous when I sat down for dinner.

"When you start the day strong, momentum will stay with you throughout the day. Remember we discussed earlier that people who eat breakfast have a much easier time not overeating at night. I thought I was doing myself a favor by not eating breakfast. But that can sabotage all your efforts because your brain really thinks you're starving by evening! That's always discouraging when you're trying your hardest to eat right and lose weight."

"Boy, don't I know it."

"Emily, after drinking your water in the morning, break the fast your body has had while sleeping by eating a healthy combination of fats, proteins, and carbs. You can make a bowl of steel cut oats (carbs) with some almonds and walnuts (fats and protein), blueberries (carbs) on top and a ½ cup of almond milk (fats and protein) and you'll be good to go. Or you could make an omelet (protein) with chicken sausage (fat and protein) and lots of veggies. There are lots of options for good eating here."

"Number 7: Pack healthy snacks and plan meals. I learned to pack snacks and plan my meals *ahead of time*. This relieved a lot of stress and kept me from falling into an intense hunger mode when I had meetings or appointments that kept me from eating on time. *Hangry* is a real phenomenon, you know? Ever been so hungry you could eat a shoe? Or an entire basket of chips at a Mexican restaurant?"

"It's like you have eyes in the back of your head!"

"I only know because I did it so many times back when I was struggling. I tried to suppress my appetite all day and then *bam*. They put a basket of chips in front of me and I was completely defenseless."

"Oh good, it's not just me."

"I was depleting myself and then became famished because I wasn't fueling my body. Once I learned how healthy snacking could help me, I lost even more weight because hunger pangs didn't control me or make me overeat. Our bodies are meant to be fueled every few hours. Our brains require a steady supply of glucose and if they get low on fuel they are quick to let us know in not-so-subtle ways. Some people get headaches, experience dizziness, or feel shaky. But almost everyone feels their mood shift a little south."

"Girl, I am telling you. I'm in the South Pole sometimes!" Emily confessed.

"Why do we fight eating when our brain is telling us it needs food?"

"Because I used to tell myself 'I'm fat and I don't deserve to eat until I'm beyond hungry.'"

Woah. Hold the phone. I didn't expect that answer. I was actually asking a rhetorical question but this obviously touched a nerve.

"Emily, you said 'used to.' What changed this and what do you tell yourself now?"

"It started to change when I understood that you came from the same place of desperation I did but you didn't make it your identity any more. Then when I did the homework assignment on I AM, it made me realize that my words are powerful and I needed to be grateful for how God made me, fearfully and wonderfully. I'm learning that I am who God says I am and that is a whole different vernacular than what I'm used to speaking over myself. But I'm getting better. Each day. Little by little."

"And that's the best kind of progress, Em! I'm so proud of you."

"I knew you would be," she replied smiling. "Now, back to those snacks. What's up with that?"

"Emily, snacking when done the wrong way—too much, too sweet, or after dinner—can make us gain weight. That's why snacking seems counterintuitive. Here's the thing: snack choices must be *clean* choices and in *small* amounts to do the trick and not get in the way of weight loss. The purpose of snacking is not to eat an entire meal. It is to keep your blood sugar balanced if you have to go several hours without eating. If you're starting the day with enough water, a breakfast with good amounts of protein and fat, and good gut health supplements, you should be able to make it 3 to 4 hours without feeling overly hungry. But let's say for example, you have breakfast at 6 a.m. and don't have lunch until noon or after. That's 6 hours without eating! You are going to need a snack to stretch that far between meals if you still want to be nice to people." Laughing, Emily raised a hand to high-five me.

I got you, girl.

"The best snacks combine all 3 food groups such as natural almond butter and fruit. A handful of almonds with *Craisins* and oats. Pumpkin seeds and cashews with low-sugar granola. Guacamole and veggies. Hummus and sliced veggies, or even hummus by itself since it contains proteins, fats, and carbs. Have snacks made ahead of time so you can easily access them. Keep a nut or seed mix in a baggie for your car, briefcase, desk, or gym bag. I make this a regular habit since one never knows when meetings will run over or the unexpected will come up."

I warned, "Don't give in to the cookies and candy at work. There's a reason co-workers bring them to work—they don't want the temptation in *their* house. Sugary treats spike your blood sugar, drop your energy like a hot potato, and make you store fat. And you're never more vulnerable than when you're overly hungry."

"Not anymore!" Emily interjected with excitement.

"Also, try to put something in your stomach before you go to a party or grocery shopping. This is a trick I learned when I was breaking free of my bad eating habits and I still practice it today. Typically the choices at parties are not particularly clean so it's best to eat a snack before you go. That will take the edge off your hunger and give you more control over your choices. If you go with some food in your stomach, it will be much easier to avoid overdoing it at the cheesecake table."

I wanted to reiterate that this was not a diet plan, but a life-style change so I urged Emily further, "The one thing that ties the Golden 7 together is *planning.* There will be a section in your planner to help you create a list of meals, complete with delicious, clean recipes. If you will invest the time to carefully plan and prepare each day, you will be amazed how much better you feel in a short amount of time. How great would that be?"

"That would be incredible!! I'm already seeing progress in my goals to…"

"…stop feeling bad, lose weight, and get some amazing energy?" I interjected.

Emily laughed, recalling our first meeting and her salty disposition. "Exactly."

"So that's my story, Em, of how I started living again. How I got my health back, lost weight, and broke the terrible chain of bad choices that kept me defeated. The process changed me physically and emotionally. The entire journey rescued me out of a very dark place and gave me the courage to hope against all odds that I would become a stronger, healthier, wiser, and better person than before."

"And…are you?" Emily asked.

"Wisdom is a muscle—the more you flex it the stronger you become. The stronger you become on the inside, the more it shows on the outside. In the beginning, it was really difficult to transform my heart and head to make the necessary effort that would get me to where I wanted to go. But I was so tired of always feeling guilty and ashamed I was ready to bear the burden of discipline to become a better me. I'd finally had enough of my old ways and I was ready to do whatever was needed to be new. Sometimes what we know the best feels comfortable, almost like an old friend, but it can be a chain that holds us prisoner to our habits. I learned to keep rising, reaching for a new level, even after falling hard. Nothing could stop me. I wanted extraordinary, not ordinary."

"Wow! I want to rise to a new level too! You've been committed to yours for a long time now without yo-yo-ing back and forth after every disappointment. If you had to narrow it down to one thing—one first step that kept propelling you forward—what would you say it was?"

"It *was* and still *is*—crying out to God for help. Through a lot of prayer—and I mean, a *lot* of prayer—He gave me these tools to get free and stay free for the rest of my life. The more I exercised my wisdom muscle through living this plan, the stronger I became in all areas of my life, but it was God's love that saved me from myself."

"And now look at you!" Emily exclaimed. "You've taken a stubborn cynic like me and infused energy into these dry bones through those same tools. You've got me doing things I never dreamed of like praying, hiking, jumping Double Dutch, eating spinach salads with flax and EVOO!" Emily said laughing. Then turning serious, Emily unflinchingly proclaimed, "And as much as I usually hate being wrong, I'm happy to say, this time I was completely wrong. This whole process has changed me from the inside out. Listen to this," she proudly announced, pulling her I AM assignment out of her pocket.

"I am a fearless warrior!

"I am a disciplined person!

"I speak life and love over others!

"I conquer the insurmountable challenges in front of me!

"I am exceedingly strong and courageous!

"I have extraordinary energy for all my work!

"I am positioned for miraculous success!

"I am a daughter of the King and I am stepping into my destiny!"

"Diamond Head, here I come!" she declared, raising her first in triumph!

I literally couldn't speak and was jumping for joy inside.

And we danced and celebrated in the hallway where chains had been broken, impossible dreams had been born, and the loftiest mountains were about to be conquered.

"Nothing, not even a mighty mountain will stand in your way."
Zechariah 4:6,7

Reach Laurie

For speaking engagements go to:
book.laurieellsworth@gmail.com

For more information on natural, plant-based gut health supplements or to order go to:

Plexusworldwide.com/laurieellsworth

Decide, Plan & Begin

Hi there, friend!

Boy do we have a LOT in common! You picked up this book because you, like Emily, are ready for change and excited to embrace the tools you'll need to be your very best. I'm excited for that too! You want to feel like a million bucks with amazing and vibrant energy. More enthusiasm. More confidence. You want to get rid of the old habits that are keeping you stuck. You're ready to step out in courage and commit to a plan that will have a lasting impact on your waistline, health, dreams, and future. Yep, we're on the same journey toward living at an EXTRAORDINARY level. I love that we're doing this together. You're done settling for less than your best—living with ordinary habits, ordinary energy, and ordinary expectations. Glory! Me too!

I used to settle—and it never felt good. Ever. It's *easy* to settle. The old person in us wants to keep us there. And that voice can be *very* convincing.

You're healthy enough. Why do you need to work out when you're already so busy? A salad? You'll be hungry in two hours! You're mostly pretty healthy, and waaaaaay better than a lot of other people you know. You're fine. Trust me.

But we know deep down in our hearts we're definitely not where we want to be. There's a much higher level we can reach. A level where we embrace new tools, even though they make us uncomfortable. A level where we make hard decisions that make us stronger instead of defaulting to familiar choices that keep us stuck. A level where our clothes fit loosely and we feel terrific. A level where we have a great night of sleep and wake up ready to conquer the world. Or at least our little section of it. A level where we say kind things to ourselves, declare who we are and who we're becoming. A level where we forget what it feels like to feel awful.

Easy doesn't give you any of those.

Easy makes pronouncements against hard choices and a mindset of excellence. *Easy* justifies a way out of commitment. "Boy, work has exhausted me lately. A glass of wine is what I need tonight, not a workout." *Easy* whispers against discipline. "Man, I'm hungry. What does it matter if I eat this one cookie? I've been good all week. At least I'm having a diet soda to balance it." But easy doesn't *feel* right. Easy promises short term peace but furnishes long term pain. The chirping in my own ear used to say, *you deserve to relax. You deserve that cookie. You deserve to put your feet up, take life easy, get lost in social media. You deserve to comfort yourself with whatever sounds good.*

You deserve. Who really can argue with that? We *do* work hard so what's wrong with skipping a daily workout? Life is stressful so how can a small bowl of ice cream hurt us, right? But "easy" isn't giving us what we really want. To feel better. Look better. And live better.

Friend, what you *deserve* is built from awesome decisions and a fierce resolve that doesn't make excuses. At the end of the day you want what comes from better choices which is infinitely more rewarding and will ultimately take you where you want to go. You got some mountains in the way? Not to worry. We got a mountain-mover who goes before and behind us, holding victory in his right hand.

DECIDING

SO WHAT IS IT YOU WANT? First, and foremost—you have to decide what is most important to you. Deciding what is "your best you" is the first step toward life-changing health. So what does that look like? What do you truly want? Once you determine that, your decision becomes your goal. Zig Ziglar used to say, "A goal properly set is halfway reached." So true, Zig. So let's set a goal that lights a fire. A goal that is big and exciting and a little scary. A goal that fans a flame in your entire soul and fuels a bonfire in your heart!

Setting the results you want and working towards them every

day with the right tools will do more to guarantee your success than any other factor!

We know our thoughts create the conditions of our lives. Our thoughts dictate how we spend our time. Our thoughts determine the habits that propel us forward or keep us defeated. So we must spend a little bit of time disciplining ourselves to think about what it is we REALLY WANT and how we can achieve it. This will greatly increase the chances of our goals becoming a reality since it forces our brains to engage in a new process of priority and achievement.

PLANNING

Writing that goal is the next step, and it is powerful. This is a "psycho-neuro-motor activity." As a result, you firmly set your goal into your subconscious mind which the brain then works on 24/7 to make a reality.

Turns out there is a phenomenal way to write down your goals, similar to the SMART version that acts like a personal assistant in your subconscious—always reminding you what you should be working on. Answer the following 4 questions and you will be well on your way towards "setting a goal that excites your brain" and having what you want.

1. WHAT? Decide what it is you really want to achieve in detail. The more defined the goal, the better.
2. WHEN? Decide when you will accomplish your goals. Give them a deadline.
3. WHY? What's the motive behind what you want? Usually the "why" is connected to how you want to feel. Make it compelling. Let your heart lead you. This has a very influential effect on your commitment. If you don't know your "why," it becomes much easier to blow off the habits and actions that will get you there. Your WHY will firm up your commitment to follow through on the work it will take to achieve your goal.
4. HOW? Then write down how you're going to get there—what tools and actions are you going to use to achieve your goals?

Here are some tips to sharpen this exercise. If you just say, "I want to lose weight" that doesn't excite your brain or incite any kind of commitment in your heart. It's way too vague. Instead, say something like, "I want to lose 10 pounds of fat in 30 days because I really want to look better in my favorite clothes! Or "I want to lose 20 pounds so I can have more energy." I will accomplish this when I use these tools daily—water, a thankful list, gut health supplements, CLEAN eating, sleep, and exercise."

Then you can know you have a clear picture of where you going and how to get there.

The next step is to make a contract with yourself with those goals. Contracts connote a weight of importance to your brain which increases your chance of actually accomplishing your goal. Statistics tell us that people who write down their goals with a signed contract have an **80% greater success rate** than those who do not write them down. This tells your brain you're achieving something important and all through the day it will remind you to accomplish it.

Your brain will not initially like the idea of new actions. It seems to prefer routine over change. That's why there's a certain level of uncertainty or even fear when you think about changing what you eat or adding supplements or exercise to your daily schedule. That's why writing down your goals is important to give your brain a subliminal alarm. Yes, your brain reminds you with a little checklist of what you said you would do. However, according to Mel Robbins, author of The 5 Second Rule, you must act on an idea—such as drinking water, exercising, or taking your supplements—within 5 seconds of when it first appears in your mind or your brain will kill it. If you hesitate in those first five seconds, the inspiration leaves completely and you don't *feel* like doing the new action any more. It's in those 5 seconds where you hear yourself say, "I've got 20 minutes for a walk," that you either do or don't take action and get yourself out the front door! If those 5 seconds pass and you don't physically act on the thought, there is a GREAT chance you won't take any action at all and that new habit will be gone like the wind. **You must intertwine the inspiration of your brain to a physical act of movement.**

This is why you can hear the most inspiring presentation and have the greatest intentions to change a habit, but the new thought quickly passes without any tangible actions being taken and those great ideas vanish into thin air. Now you don't *feel* like it. And it's virtually impossible to make yourself do something then. But if you marry your impulse to some kind of action, even if it is a brand new behavior, you create a neural pathway in your brain to keep doing that activity. There is a physical force required to change your behavior. Action begets action in a powerful way. If you wait until you feel like it, you will never do it. Never. Your brain will tap the brake to anything new because routine is safer. If you feel anxious or uncertain about new actions, your brain wants to protect you. Your feelings mess everything up! Your brain searches for the easy way out and doing something new is *not* easy. You have to force yourself to do that which will bring you the results you deeply desire. *Force* yourself to get past what you feel. *Force* yourself to be uncomfortable with a new behavior.

You have to do the things you don't want to do to have the things you really want to have!

I've seen this happen with something as simple as drinking water. I set my alarm for 6 A.M., 9 A.M., 12 P.M., 3 P.M., and 6 P.M. to remind myself to drink. But if the alarm goes off and I don't start moving toward my water bottle within 5 seconds, the thought completely leaves me. I hesitate past 5 seconds and the next thing I know, the next alarm is going off 3 hours later and I'm ridiculously thirsty. No wonder! Setting the alarm is a great plan. But the 5 second rule tells me I need to act quickly before my brain kills the idea. It feels like an inner snooze button if I don't act right away. My brain will step in and talk me out of it. And it seems true every time.

BEGINNING

Lastly, track your progress. You must keep Top of the Mind Awareness —or TOMA—to succeed. What you think about the most, your brain will make happen. If TOMA didn't have a huge amount of influence on your brain, companies wouldn't spend millions of dollars on a 30-second commercial that you see over and over. It works! Use this to your advantage to achieve your goals. If you don't thing about what you want every day, guess what? It's a guarantee you won't achieve it because the busyness of life will derail you. If you do, you will. It's a proven fact.

Zig Ziglar said 'You have to "be" before you can "do", and do before you can "have".' It's so true, friend. We can't do the same things each day and expect to have different results. That has never worked in the past and it's guaranteed to never work in your future. This health journey is about **be**ing committed to **do** simple actions so you can **have** a healthier, stronger, better you. When you rise out of ordinary decisions you will see yourself rise to a new level of extraordinary goals. That is when you will become unstoppable in every aspect of your life!!!

"First we make our habits.
Then our habits make us." ~ John Dryden

Plan Tomorrow Beginning Tonight

Most of your success, both now and in the future, will be accomplished on the **front side of each day.** If you want to leap out of the gates on Monday morning ready to conquer the world, you have to prepare on *Sunday night.* Once Monday arrives, it becomes a mad dash to stay up with the whirlwind of life. Your best days will happen when you prepare and plan what you will eat, drink, how and when you will exercise, and what bedtime rituals you will include, BEFORE they happen!! Because guess what? If you don't prepare and plan at least the day before, there's a good chance your healthy habits won't happen. There will be unexpected fires to put out almost on a daily basis, which means your awesome new habits could go right out the window. Carefully prepare the day before. Or even the weekend before. Repeat. Prepare. Repeat. This is the key to your success.

If you just let life happen to you, it will be almost impossible to rise out of your current situation. Take control by planning ahead and watch how much your health improves! Plan. Prepare. Repeat. That will help guarantee your follow through each day.

Use the following actions to help organize your food for the week.
1. Keep your water bottle full, in the frig ready to grab! Set your alarm to drink every 3 hours until you automatically remember.

2. Make a large spinach salad for the week ahead. Lots of veggies, nuts, seeds, and eggs on top. Try to start every meal with a dark green salad with balsamic dressing. (Recipe section).

3. Make Hard-boiled eggs. This is a great snack to pop into your mouth in between meals. I use a tiny bit of Avocado mayo on top. I've included instruction for how to make perfect hard-

boiled eggs every time and it works like a charm. Make them on the weekends and they'll be easy to grab through the week.

4. Make up a nut mixture of your favorite nuts, excluding peanuts since they don't offer as much nutritional value. Use almonds, walnuts, pecans, macadamias, and cashews and add to a pretty glass jar. Keep this on your kitchen counter so you can grab a handful to stave off hunger. You can also put this on your salads.

5. Make a smoothie of spinach, water, chia and flax seeds (always the milled kind), coconut oil, kefir or Greek yogurt, blueberries or whatever fruit you like. It's important to add the coconut oil to give it a good fat. And the Kefir adds a bit of probiotic, which is always a goal. Just put it all together, add a lid and keep in the fridge until morning. The next day, blend it in the morning for a few seconds. Walla! Easy-peasy.

6. Make up some guacamole which is full of potassium! This is a great option instead of a salad to start dinner. It's full of good fat. Just make sure you limit yourself to about 10 chips or use veggies to dip. Here's a tip, if you don't have all the ingredients you need, you can always add organic salsa to the mashed up avocado to flavor it. Yum!

7. Grill up several chicken breasts to use for salads and in dishes.

8. Make your Plexus Pink drink ready and keep it in the fridge, so it's cold and easy to grab in the morning. Set supplements on counter next to the coffee pot.

Plan—plan—plan! That is the key to changing habits without becoming overwhelmed.

Contract of Commitment

So what is a goal you want to accomplish? There may be several, but let's start with one for 30 days and then you can tackle other goals after you've accomplished this one.

WHAT—I want to become:

_____

_____

WHEN—by this date:

_____

_____

WHY—because I will feel:

_____

_____

My biggest obstacle in the past has been:

_____

_____

_____

How will you use the 5 tools as actions?

Water_____
Thankful
List_____
Exercise_____
Eating CLEAN_____

I,_____, agree to work toward this healthy goal and in doing so, comply with the terms and dates of this contract.

Signature: Date:

Witness: Date:

To help me even more with TOMA, I have the following sentences written on a piece of paper on my fridge:

I WANT TO LOSE 8 POUNDS in 30 days BECAUSE I FEEL so much better when my clothes fit well!!!

The awesome actions I will take EACH DAY to accomplish this are:

List my blessings to nurture a spirit of gratitude. Send this to my husband each day.

Drink water every 3 hours. Set my alarm since I know I will get busy and forget.

Healthy bedtime rituals for better sleep and sweet dreams. Chamomile tea, prayer, and reading at 9 PM.

Walk and stretch daily to keep strong muscles and joints. Schedule group classes on my calendar!

Eat CLEAN foods that are one ingredient to fuel my body. Plan ahead for meals, recipes, and shopping.

Take plant-based supplements to strengthen my gut health.

What will you put on YOUR Frig? Type it out below. Print it. Get it on your fridge or bathroom mirror. Think about it daily. Watch it become a REALITY!

I AM

This is your I AM assignment. After the I AM fill in who you want to become in one line sentences with as many as you can think of. This will become your new script that you say to yourself every single day. And you know what? The more you say it, the more you will believe it and that will change your life! You're not who you were. You're not where you've been. You are who God says you are. You are who he has created you to be. You have a calling in front of you that only you can answer.

So here you go, friend. Xo

I AM:

Recipes

Delicious Vinaigrette

Ingredients
¼ c. balsamic vinegar (I use pomegranate-flavored)
1 t. fresh lemon juice
1 t. minced garlic
1 t. onions, minced (opt.)
1 T. Dijon mustard
2/3 c. EVOO (Extra Virgin Olive Oil)
Herbs, salt, and pepper to taste.

Directions
1. Whisk together vinegar, lemon juice, garlic, onions, mustard, herbs, and salt and pepper.
2. Slowly pour olive oil into the mixture while whisking vigorously. This will emulsify it so it stays blended.
3. Pour into jar. Shake well before using.

I use this on literally everything from salads to roasted veggies to baked potatoes to steak. Simply delish on everything from salads to roasted veggies to steak.

Perfect Hard-boiled Eggs

Ingredients
1 dozen farm fresh eggs

Directions
1. Boil water in large pot. Make sure it is a rolling boil.
2. Reduce the heat to a mild boil. Carefully add a dozen eggs. I use a large ladle to set them in the boiling water.
3. Cook on mild boil for 14 minutes. (Use a timer)
4. Drain and let eggs sit in an ice bath for 8 minutes.
5. Peel all the eggs (skin should slip right off) and store in glass container in frig. Walla! How easy is that! Wished I had known this 20 years ago!

Bircher Muesli

Ingredients
1 cup of yogurt
1 cup of milk (Kefir or coconut milk) I recently switched to Kefir since it's a probiotic)
1 T. vanilla
1 cup of (organic) Oats
1 cup of organic blueberries
1 organic apple, chopped to bite size, with skin
1 cup of nuts (I like sliced almonds or walnuts)
Optional: 1 t. cinnamon and you can also add a drop or two of liquid Stevia for sweetness

Directions
1. Mix all the liquids plus vanilla.
2. Add oats and mix.
3. Add the apple, blueberries, and nuts.
4. Set in frig overnight. Stays good for several days.

There is no wrong way to make this. You can easily double this for a larger family. If you like more nuts or want to add something else, make it your own. The nuts give it the protein and fat.

Spinach smoothie (in a blender, Bullet, or Vitamix):

Ingredients
2 cups spinach
½ cup blueberries
1 T. flax seed (make sure it's milled)
1 T. Chia seeds
1 heaping T. coconut oil or coconut Kefir
1 cup liquid kefir
1-2 cups of water (depending on how thick you like it.)

Directions
1. Blend and walla!!

Recipes

Black Bean Breakfast Bowl

Ingredients
4-5 eggs
Avocado oil or coconut oil
Black beans
Avocado
Salsa

Directions
1. Scramble 4-5 eggs in avocado oil or coconut oil (my favorite)
2. Heat up 1 cup of black beans.
3. Place ½ cup of black beans in bottom of 2 bowls.
4. Add cooked eggs on top.
5. Top the eggs with ½ sliced avocado each bowl.
6. Finish the top with ½ cup salsa or to taste.

Coconut Power Balls

Ingredients
½ c. natural Almond Butter
1/8 c. honey
1 T. vanilla
½ c. unsweetened shredded coconut
1 T. chia seeds
1 T. milled flax seed
½ c. rolled oats
1 T. chocolate Chips
1/3 c. protein powder (optional)

Directions
1. In large bowl, mix the almond butter, honey, and vanilla.
2. Add in coconut, flax, chia, oats, and chocolate chips.
3. Add in optional protein powder.
4. Use your hands to mix and work into balls.
5. If it is too dry add a drop more of honey or if it is too gooey add more oats or coconut. These can be stored in the refrigerator for a week or a freezer for a month. Great healthy treat for a party!

Homemade Taco Seasoning

Ingredients
1 teaspoons chili powder
1 ½ t. paprika
1 t. onion powder
½ t. sea salt
½ t. garlic powder
½ t. ground cumin
½ t. oregano
¼ t. freshly ground black pepper or to taste
1 pinch cayenne pepper (optional)
1 pinch red pepper flakes (optional)

Directions
1. Mix chili powder, paprika, onion powder, sea salt, garlic powder, cumin, oregano, black pepper, cayenne pepper, and red pepper flakes in a bowl.
2. Add to browning meat when meat is partially browned. After browned completely, add 1/2 to 1 cup water and cook down to blend flavors.
3. Add to salad and top with small amounts of yogurt or sour cream (not reduced fat type), or fill taco shells and top with tomatoes and spinach or kale. (small amounts of cheese are fine.)

Homemade Hummus

Ingredients
2 cans chickpeas, drained (save liquid)
¼ C. EVOO
2 T. minced garlic or 2 cloves minced
2 T. tahini (sesame paste found in organic aisle)
1 r. ground cumin
Juice of 1 lemon

Directions
1. Mix in blender or Vitamix.
2. Add some of the chickpea liquid for desire thickness. I usually end of adding about ½ cup back in.

Mini Sausage Quiche

Ingredients
1 package of Adelle's Chicken and apple sausage, chopped bite size
1 t. avocado oil
8 ounces mushrooms, chopped small
¼ cup sliced scallions
¼ cup shredded Pepper Jack (or your cheese choice)
1 teaspoon freshly ground pepper
7 eggs
1 cup milk (try almond if you don't want your eggs to taste coconuty.)

Directions
1. Position rack in center of oven; preheat to 325°F. Coat a nonstick muffin tin generously with organic spray.
2. Heat a large nonstick skillet over medium-high heat.
3. Add sausage and cook until golden brown, 6 to 8 minutes.
4. Transfer to a bowl to cool, and then crumble in small pieces.
5. Add oil to the pan. Add mushrooms and cook, stirring often, until golden brown, 5 to 7 minutes.
6. Transfer mushrooms to the bowl with the sausage.
7. Let cool for 5 minutes.
8. Stir in scallions, cheese and pepper.
9. Whisk eggs and milk in a medium bowl.
10. Divide the egg mixture evenly among the prepared muffin cups.
11. Sprinkle a heaping tablespoon of the sausage mixture into each cup.
12. Bake until the tops are just beginning to brown, 25 minutes.
13. Let cool for 5 minutes.
14. Place a rack on top of the pan, flip it over and turn the quiches out onto the rack. Turn upright and let cool completely.

Salsa Chicken

Ingredients
1 cup salsa, your choice from the organic aisle
1 t. cumin
1 t. chili powder
1 T. fresh lime juice
1 pound skinless, boneless chicken breasts
Fresh cilantro, chopped

Directions

1. Preheat oven to 375 °F.
2. Combine first 4 ingredients.
3. Spray baking dish with organic spray.
4. Place chicken on top.
5. Pour salsa mixture over chicken, and then flip the chicken to coat it well with salsa mix.
6. Bake 20-30 minutes.
7. Test chicken for doneness. Try not to overbake but you don't want it pink either.
8. Be sure to baste chicken occasionally with salsa mix during the baking process. Top with fresh cilantro. Walla!!! Delicioso.

Grocery List

Try a grocery list like this—or make up your own healthy version. These quantities are for 2-4 people for two weeks.

ALL ORGANIC PRODUCE:
Large container of fresh spinach or Kale (prewashed)
Your choice of vegetables: peppers, mushrooms, broccoli, onion, cauliflower, cucumbers, asparagus, etc. (deep colors)
4 avocadoes
Minced garlic
Bag of lemons, bag of limes
Sweet potatoes
Red potatoes
Blueberries, blackberries, raspberries, strawberries (you pick farms or farmer's market even better)
Pineapples, mangoes, cherries

How to wash produce: When you get your produce from the store, wash it in a big bowl of water and vinegar (50% of each) for 10 minutes (gets rid of parasites, bacteria, pesticides). Then you can easily grab it out of the fridge to eat.

DAIRY AISLE:
Plain Greek yogurt (low sugar, **FULL fat**). Try to find less than 10 gm of sugar
Kerry gold butter
Coconut milk
Farm fresh eggs— (I use 3 dozen in 2 weeks)

SEEDS/NUTS:
Walnuts, almonds, pecans, cashews (unless you have peanut allergies)
Pumpkin seeds or sunflower seeds (hulled)

BAKING AISLE:
Best real vanilla
Old-fashioned oats and/or steel cut
Ground flax seeds
Ground Chia seeds
Balsamic vinegar

Extra virgin olive oil, cold-pressed (cooking with low heat)
Avocado oil (cooking with high heat)
Coconut oil, virgin, cold-pressed, unrefined (smoothies and cooking with medium to high heat)

MEAT: ALL ORGANIC
Turkey
2 packages of free-range chicken breasts
Adelle's chicken and apple sausage
Ground Chuck
Steak (whatever cut you like)
Salmon wild-caught

OTHER:
Almond butter (or make your own at the grocery store)
Lower sugar tomato sauce (I like Muir Glen)
Gluten free pasta or zoodles (zucchini noodles)
Chicken broth (2 large containers)
Garbanzo Beans (for the Hummus recipe)
Low sugar salsa
Blue chips or non-grain chips
Dave's Bread (not GF, but a superb choice if you do wheat) or any gluten free
Local honey

Eating Out

Here are some tips to ensure you stay on track when you eat out. Eating out can often be a deal breaker to your success and your best laid plans because the portion sizes are usually gargantuan.

1. Have 2 glasses of water before the meal. Helps keep you from overeating because you're thirsty.
2. Always start with a spinach salad or dark green salad. Fill up on awesome veggies full of antioxidants while you're hungry.
3. Order only GRILLED meat and veggies, not meat with breading. Breading is usually full of processed white flour which grows bad bacteria.
4. Split the entrée if possible. Portion sizes these days are gargantuan.
5. No dessert. Fill up on foods that will fuel you instead of releasing insulin that promotes fat storage.
6. Do NOT eat after dinner. These are calories you don't need and it can interfere with sleep.
7. Limit alcohol. Wine and beer are full of sugar which grows bad bacteria and can also interrupt sleep.

Use the 1/3 RULE: Fats, carbs, proteins. Make sure your plate has plenty of good fats, protein, and carbs in the form of veggies, not grains. Skip the rolls before dinner. There's a reason they're free.

NO sweeteners (except liquid stevia), NO soda, NO diet products, NO white flour, NO processed sugar, high-processed ice creams, sugary sauce of any kind. All of these KILL good bacteria and help bad bacteria grow! Inflammation is the result of too much bad bacteria, which causes a whole mess of issues in your body, excruciating pain, and keeps you from losing weight.

Clean eating requires a lot of chewing to break down the food. Your meals will take longer but food with fiber helps you feel full longer and stimulates quick elimination. You won't even want dessert.

Health Habit Checklist

Y_____ N_____ 1. I get at least 7 hours of sleep on most nights.

Y_____ N_____ 2. I eat breakfast most mornings.

Y_____ N_____ 3. I drink at least 8 glasses (8 oz. each) of water on most days.

Y_____ N_____ 4. I eat at least 4 servings of vegetables on most days.

Y_____ N_____ 5. I eat at least 3 servings of protein on most days.

Y_____ N_____ 6. I get at least 10 minutes of sunlight on most days.

Y_____ N_____ 7. I exercise aerobically at least 5 days a week.

Y_____ N_____ 8. I lift weights at least twice a week.

Y_____ N_____ 9. I stretch for at least 10 minutes on most days.

Y_____ N_____ 10. I have regular bedtime habits that help reduce stress.

Health Habit Journal

Today's Date:

God is for me and I will succeed! These are my awesome actions today:

WATER

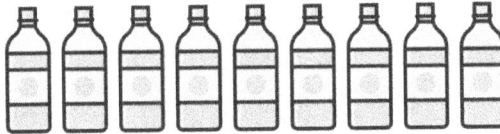

CLEAN Eating (fat, protein, veggie carbs):

Breakfast:

Lunch:

Dinner:

PLAY (exercise):

Bedtime Rituals and Sleep:

Gut Health Supplements:

TODAY I am thankful for:

"Giving thanks is a sacrifice that truly honors me."
Psalm 50:23

<u>Leaving these requests and concerns with you, Lord:</u>

Health Habit Journal

Today's Date:

God is for me and I will succeed! These are the awesome actions I used today:

WATER

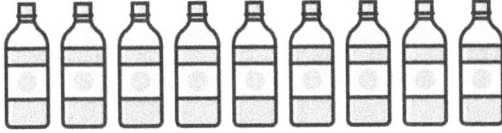

CLEAN Eating (fat, protein, veggie carbs):

Breakfast:

Lunch:

Dinner:

Supplements:

PLAY (exercise):

Sleep:

Poop:

Rituals:

TODAY I am thankful for:

"Blessings chase the righteous."
Proverbs 13:21

<u>Leaving these concerns with you, Lord:</u>

Health Habit Journal

Today's Date:

God is for me and I will succeed! These are the awesome actions I used today:

WATER

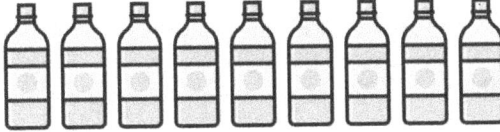

CLEAN Eating (fat, protein, veggie carbs):

Breakfast:

Lunch:

Dinner:

Supplements:

PLAY (exercise):

Sleep:

Poop:

Rituals:

TODAY I am thankful for:

"Do not fear anything except the Lord Almighty. He alone is the Holy
One. If you fear him, you need fear nothing else."
Isaiah 8:13

<u>Leaving these concerns with you, Lord:</u>

Health Habit Journal

Today's Date:

God is for me and I will succeed! These are the awesome actions I used today:

WATER

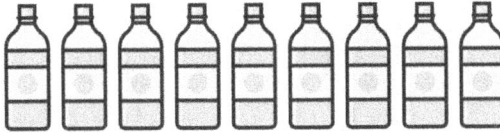

CLEAN Eating (fat, protein, veggie carbs):

Breakfast:

Lunch:

Dinner:

Supplements:

PLAY (exercise):

Sleep:

Poop:

Rituals:

TODAY I am thankful for:

"Do not despise small beginnings,
for the Lord rejoices to see the work begin."
Zechariah 4:10

<u>Leaving these concerns with you, Lord:</u>

Health Habit Journal

Today's Date:

God is for me and I will succeed! These are the awesome actions I used today:

WATER

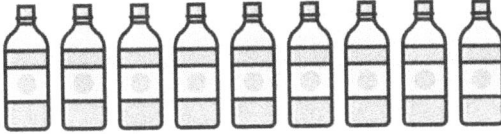

CLEAN Eating (fat, protein, veggie carbs):

Breakfast:

Lunch:

Dinner:

Supplements:

PLAY (exercise):

Sleep:

Poop:

Rituals:

TODAY I am thankful for:

"NOW I will rescue you and make you a symbol
and a source of blessing! So don't be afraid or discouraged,
instead get on with your work."
Zechariah 8:13

<u>Leaving these concerns with you, Lord:</u>

Health Habit Journal

Today's Date:

God is for me and I will succeed! These are the awesome actions I used today:

WATER

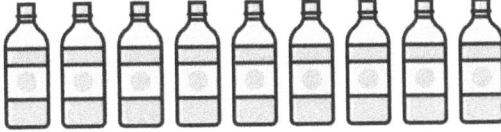

CLEAN Eating (fat, protein, veggie carbs):

Breakfast:

Lunch:

Dinner:

Supplements:

PLAY (exercise):

Sleep:

Poop:

Rituals:

TODAY I am thankful for:

"Seek first the kingdom of God and His righteousness
and all these things will be added to you."
Matthew 6:33

Leaving these concerns with you, Lord:

Health Habit Journal

Today's Date:

God is for me and I will succeed! These are the awesome actions I used today:

WATER

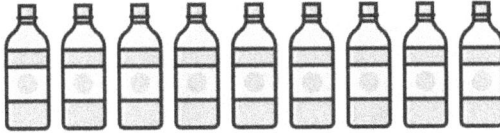

CLEAN Eating (fat, protein, veggie carbs):

Breakfast:

Lunch:

Dinner:

Supplements:

PLAY (exercise):

Sleep:

Poop:

Rituals:

TODAY I am thankful for:

"The most important piece of clothing you must wear is love."
Colossians 3:14

Leaving these concerns with you, Lord:

Health Habit Journal

Today's Date:

God is for me and I will succeed! These are the awesome actions I used today:

WATER

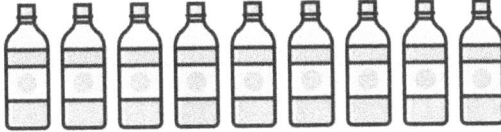

CLEAN Eating (fat, protein, veggie carbs):

Breakfast:

Lunch:

Dinner:

Supplements:

PLAY (exercise):

Sleep:

Poop:

Rituals:

TODAY I am thankful for:

"Let love be your highest goal."
I Corinthians 14:1

<u>Leaving these concerns with you, Lord:</u>

Health Habit Journal

Today's Date:

God is for me and I will succeed! These are the awesome actions I used today:

WATER

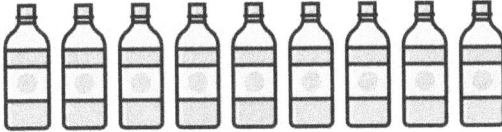

CLEAN Eating (fat, protein, veggie carbs):

Breakfast:

Lunch:

Dinner:

Supplements:

PLAY (exercise):

Sleep:

Poop:

Rituals:

TODAY I am thankful for:

"For you are the fountain of life, the light by which we see."
Psalm 36:9

<u>Leaving these concerns with you, Lord:</u>

Health Habit Journal

Today's Date:

God is for me and I will succeed! These are the awesome actions I used today:

WATER

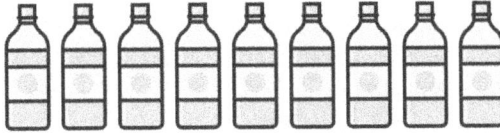

CLEAN Eating (fat, protein, veggie carbs):

Breakfast:

Lunch:

Dinner:

Supplements:

PLAY (exercise):

Sleep:

Poop:

Rituals:

TODAY I am thankful for:

"I will give you back your health and heal your wounds, says the Lord."
Jeremiah 30:17

Leaving these concerns with you, Lord:

Health Habit Journal

Today's Date:

God is for me and I will succeed! These are the awesome actions I used today:

WATER

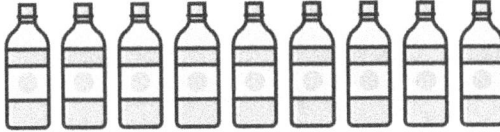

CLEAN Eating (fat, protein, veggie carbs):

Breakfast:

Lunch:

Dinner:

Supplements:

PLAY (exercise):

Sleep:

Poop:

Rituals:

TODAY I am thankful for:

"You have restored my health and have allowed me to live!"
Isaiah 38:16

Leaving these concerns with you, Lord:

Health Habit Journal

Today's Date:

God is for me and I will succeed! These are the awesome actions I used today:

WATER

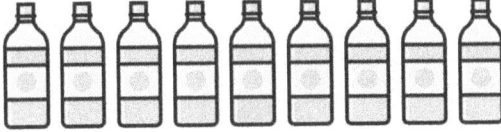

CLEAN Eating (fat, protein, veggie carbs):

Breakfast:

Lunch:

Dinner:

Supplements:

PLAY (exercise):

Sleep:

Poop:

Rituals:

TODAY I am thankful for:

"You will gain renewed health and vitality."
Proverbs 3:8

Leaving these concerns with you, Lord:

Health Habit Journal

Today's Date:

God is for me and I will succeed! These are the awesome actions I used today:

WATER

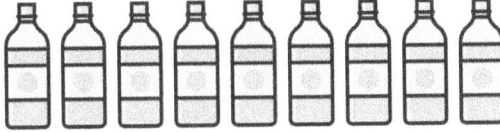

CLEAN Eating (fat, protein, veggie carbs):

Breakfast:

Lunch:

Dinner:

Supplements:

PLAY (exercise):

Sleep:

Poop:

Rituals:

TODAY I am thankful for:

"You keep track of all my sorrows.
You have collected all my tears in your bottle.
You have recorded each one in your book."
Psalm 56:8

<u>Leaving these concerns with you, Lord:</u>

Health Habit Journal

Today's Date:

God is for me and I will succeed! These are the awesome actions I used today:

WATER

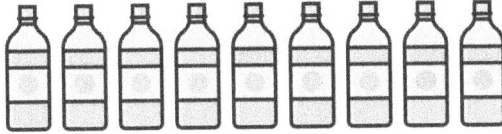

CLEAN Eating (fat, protein, veggie carbs):

Breakfast:

Lunch:

Dinner:

Supplements:

PLAY (exercise):

Sleep:

Poop:

Rituals:

TODAY I am thankful for:

"O Lord my God, I cried out to you for help,
and you restored my health."
Psalm 30:2,3

Leaving these concerns with you, Lord:

Health Habit Journal

Today's Date:

God is for me and I will succeed! These are the awesome actions I used today:

WATER

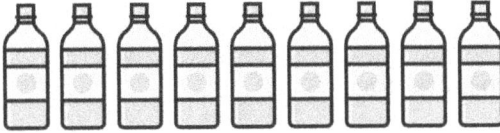

CLEAN Eating (fat, protein, veggie carbs):

Breakfast:

Lunch:

Dinner:

Supplements:

PLAY (exercise):

Sleep:

Poop:

Rituals:

TODAY I am thankful for:

"Be strong and courageous. Do not be afraid or discouraged.
The Lord your God will go ahead of you.
He will neither fail you nor forsake you."
Deuteronomy 31:6

Leaving these concerns with you, Lord:

Health Habit Journal

Today's Date:

God is for me and I will succeed! These are the awesome actions I used today:

WATER

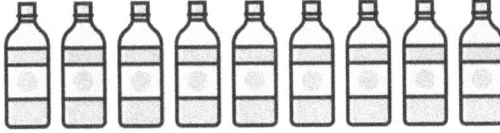

CLEAN Eating (fat, protein, veggie carbs):

Breakfast:

Lunch:

Dinner:

Supplements:

PLAY (exercise):

Sleep:

Poop:

Rituals:

TODAY I am thankful for:

"All the good things I have are from you, Lord."
Psalm 16:2

Leaving these concerns with you, Lord:

Health Habit Journal

Today's Date:

God is for me and I will succeed! These are the awesome actions I used today:

WATER

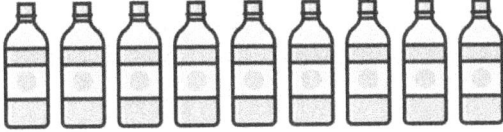

CLEAN Eating (fat, protein, veggie carbs):

Breakfast:

Lunch:

Dinner:

Supplements:

PLAY (exercise):

Sleep:

Poop:

Rituals:

TODAY I am thankful for:

"God arms me with strength; he has made my way safe."
Psalm 18:32

<u>Leaving these concerns with you, Lord:</u>

Health Habit Journal

Today's Date:

God is for me and I will succeed! These are the awesome actions I used today:

WATER

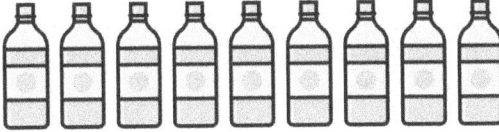

CLEAN Eating (fat, protein, veggie carbs):

Breakfast:

Lunch:

Dinner:

Supplements:

PLAY (exercise):

Sleep:

Poop:

Rituals:

TODAY I am thankful for:

"No one whose hope is in you will ever be put to shame."
Psalm 25:3

Leaving these concerns with you, Lord:

Health Habit Journal

Today's Date:

God is for me and I will succeed! These are the awesome actions I used today:

WATER

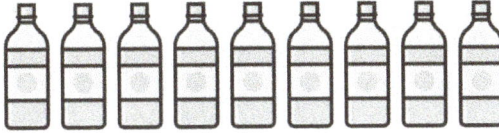

CLEAN Eating (fat, protein, veggie carbs):

Breakfast:

Lunch:

Dinner:

Supplements:

PLAY (exercise):

Sleep:

Poop:

Rituals:

TODAY I am thankful for:

"The Lord gives strength to his people;
the Lord blesses his people with peace."
Psalm 29:11

Leaving these concerns with you, Lord:

Health Habit Journal

Today's Date:

God is for me and I will succeed! These are the awesome actions I used today:

WATER

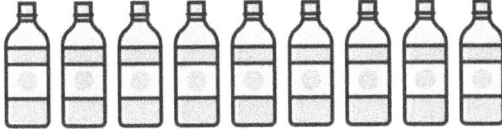

CLEAN Eating (fat, protein, veggie carbs):

Breakfast:

Lunch:

Dinner:

Supplements:

PLAY (exercise):

Sleep:

Poop:

Rituals:

TODAY I am thankful for:

"I prayed to the Lord and he answered me,
freeing me from all my fears."
Psalm 34:4

<u>Leaving these concerns with you, Lord:</u>

Health Habit Journal

Today's Date:

God is for me and I will succeed! These are the awesome actions I used today:

WATER

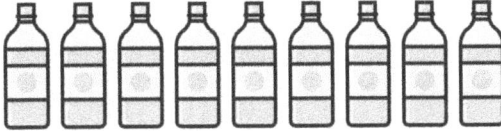

CLEAN Eating (fat, protein, veggie carbs):

Breakfast:

Lunch:

Dinner:

Supplements:

PLAY (exercise):

Sleep:

Poop:

Rituals:

TODAY I am thankful for:

"With God's help we will do mighty things."
Psalm 60:12

Leaving these concerns with you, Lord:

Health Habit Journal

Today's Date:

God is for me and I will succeed! These are the awesome actions I used today:

WATER

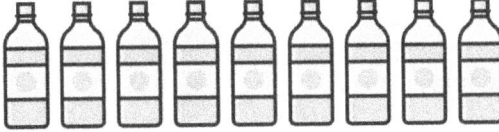

CLEAN Eating (fat, protein, veggie carbs):

Breakfast:

Lunch:

Dinner:

Supplements:

PLAY (exercise):

Sleep:

Poop:

Rituals:

TODAY I am thankful for:

"Praise the Lord; praise the God our Savior!
For each day he carries us in his arms. Our God is a God who saves!"
Psalm 68:19,20

Leaving these concerns with you, Lord:

Health Habit Journal

Today's Date:

God is for me and I will succeed! These are the awesome actions I used today:

WATER

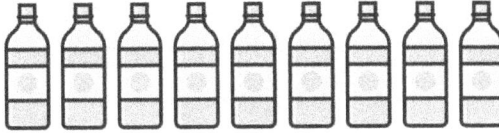

CLEAN Eating (fat, protein, veggie carbs):

Breakfast:

Lunch:

Dinner:

Supplements:

PLAY (exercise):

Sleep:

Poop:

Rituals:

TODAY I am thankful for:

"The name of the Lord is a strong tower;
the godly run to him are safe."
Proverbs 18:10

Leaving these concerns with you, Lord:

Health Habit Journal

Today's Date:

God is for me and I will succeed! These are the awesome actions I used today:

WATER

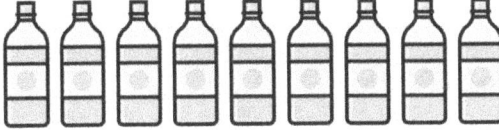

CLEAN Eating (fat, protein, veggie carbs):

Breakfast:

Lunch:

Dinner:

Supplements:

PLAY (exercise):

Sleep:

Poop:

Rituals:

TODAY I am thankful for:

"The godly may trip seven times, but each time they will rise again."
Proverbs 24.16

Leaving these concerns with you, Lord:

Health Habit Journal

Today's Date:

God is for me and I will succeed! These are the awesome actions I used today:

WATER

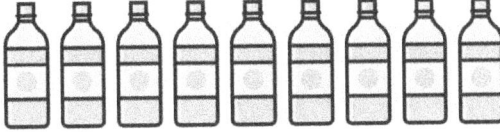

CLEAN Eating (fat, protein, veggie carbs):

Breakfast:

Lunch:

Dinner:

Supplements:

PLAY (exercise):

Sleep:

Poop:

Rituals:

TODAY I am thankful for:

"Trust in him at all times.
Pour out your heart to him,
for God is our refuge."
Psalm 62:8

Leaving these concerns with you, Lord:

Health Habit Journal

Today's Date:

God is for me and I will succeed! These are the awesome actions I used today:

WATER

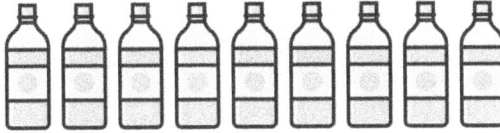

CLEAN Eating (fat, protein, veggie carbs):

Breakfast:

Lunch:

Dinner:

Supplements:

PLAY (exercise):

Sleep:

Poop:

Rituals:

TODAY I am thankful for:

"I will never forget your words,
for you have used them to restore my joy and health."
Psalm 119:93

Leaving these concerns with you, Lord:

Health Habit Journal

Today's Date:

God is for me and I will succeed! These are the awesome actions I used today:

WATER

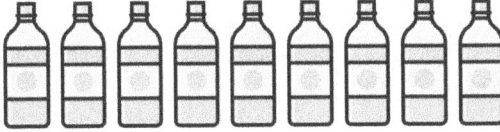

CLEAN Eating (fat, protein, veggie carbs):

Breakfast:

Lunch:

Dinner:

Supplements:

PLAY (exercise):

Sleep:

Poop:

Rituals:

TODAY I am thankful for:

"I am holding you by your right hand—
I, the Lord your God. And I say to you,
Do not be afraid. I am here to help you.
Isaiah 41:13

<u>Leaving these concerns with you, Lord:</u>

Health Habit Journal

Today's Date:

God is for me and I will succeed! These are the awesome actions I used today:

WATER

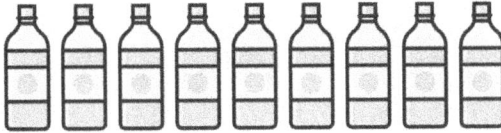

CLEAN Eating (fat, protein, veggie carbs):

Breakfast:

Lunch:

Dinner:

Supplements:

PLAY (exercise):

Sleep:

Poop:

Rituals:

TODAY I am thankful for:

"It is not by power or might, but by my Sprit says the Lord Almighty.
Nothing, not even a mountain, will stand in your way."
Zechariah 4:6,7

<u>Leaving these concerns with you, Lord:</u>

Health Habit Journal

Today's Date:

God is for me and I will succeed! These are the awesome actions I used today:

WATER

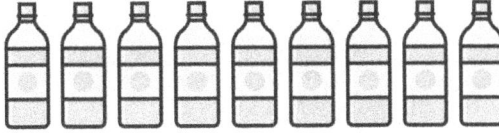

CLEAN Eating (fat, protein, veggie carbs):

Breakfast:

Lunch:

Dinner:

Supplements:

PLAY (exercise):

Sleep:

Poop:

Rituals:

TODAY I am thankful for:

"Now thanks be to God who always causes us to triumph in Christ."
II Corinthians 2:14

<u>Leaving these concerns with you, Lord:</u>

Health Habit Journal

Today's Date:

God is for me and I will succeed! These are the awesome actions I used today:

WATER

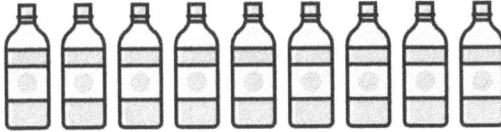

CLEAN Eating (fat, protein, veggie carbs):

Breakfast:

Lunch:

Dinner:

Supplements:

PLAY (exercise):

Sleep:

Poop:

Rituals:

TODAY I am thankful for:

"Be strong in the Lord's mighty power."
Ephesians 6:10

Leaving these concerns with you, Lord:

Health Habit Journal

Today's Date:

God is for me and I will succeed! These are the awesome actions I used today:

WATER

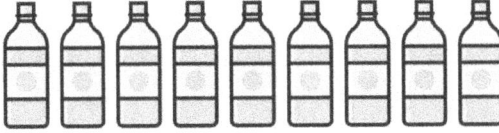

CLEAN Eating (fat, protein, veggie carbs):

Breakfast:

Lunch:

Dinner:

Supplements:

PLAY (exercise):

Sleep:

Poop:

Rituals:

TODAY I am thankful for:

"I waited patiently for the Lord to help me and he turned to me and heard my cry. He lifted me out of the pit of despair, out of the mud and mire, and set my feet on his solid rock, steadying my as I walked along. He's given me a new song to sing, a hymn of praise to our God. And many will see what he has done and be astounded, and they will put their trust in him."
Psalm 40:1-3

<u>Leaving these concerns with you, Lord:</u>

Book Recommendations

Feed Your Heart

The Bible, God. (I like the New King James or the New Living translations.)

Unashamed, Drop the baggage, pick up your freedom, fulfill your destiny, Christine Caine, Zondervan, 2016.

Jesus Calling, Morning and Evening, Sarah Young, Thomas Nelson, 2015.

Believing God, Beth Moore, Broadman and Holman, 2015.

Unglued, Making wise choice in the midst of raw emotions, Lysa Terkeurst, Zondervan, 2012.

The Circle Maker, Mark Batterson, Zondervan, 2011.

Let the Journey Begin, Finding God's best for your life, Max Lucado, Thomas Nelson, 2015

Feed your Mind

Think and Eat Yourself Smart, Dr. Caroline Leaf, Baker Books, 2016.

Switch on your Brain, Dr. Caroline Leaf, Baker Books, 2013.

Made to Crave, Lysa Terkeurst, Zondervan 2011.

Let Hope In, 4 choices that will change your life forever, Pete Wilson, Thomas

Nelson, 2013.

Dream Giver, Following your God-given destiny, Multnomah, 2003.

Breaking Busy, How to find peace and purpose in a world of crazy, Zondervan, 2016.

Battlefield of the Mind, Joyce Meyer, Warner Faith, 2002.

Feed Your Body
Eat Fat, Get Thin, Why the fat we eat is the key to sustained weight loss and vibrant health, Mark Hyman, MD. Little, Brown, and Company, 2016.

Why Diets Make Us Fat, The unintended consequences of our obsession with weight loss, Sandra Aamodt, Ph.D. 2016.

Bibliography

Chapter 1

[1]Kravitz, Len, Ph.D. *Water: The Science of Nature's Most Important Nutrient.* Retrieved from https://www.unm.edu/~lkravitz/Article%20folder/WaterUNM.html

[2]Mayo Clinic Staff. *Water: How much should you drik every day?* Retrieved from http://www.mayoclinic.org/healthy-lifestyle/nutrition-and-healthy-eating/in-depth/water/art-20044256

[3]Hazell, Kyrsty. (2012, February) *Mild Dehydration Causes Anger, Fatigue and Mood Swings, Study Reveals.* Retrieved from http://www.huffingtonpost.co.uk/2012/02/20/mild-dehydration-causes-a_n_1288964.html

[4]Consumer Reports. *Tension Headache Treatment and Prevention. A few simple steps like drinking water and doing neck exercises can relieve your pain.* Retrieved from http://www.consumerreports.org/pain-relief/tension-headache-treatment-prevention/

[5]DeFina, Dr. Laura. *Dehydration and Its Effects on Brain Health and Function.* Retrieved from http://cooperaerobics.com/Health-Tips/Prevention-Plus/Effects-of-Dehydration-on-the-Body-and-Brain.aspx

Chapter 3

[1]Jones, Jeffrey. M. *In U.S., 40% Get Less Than Recommended Amount of Sleep.* Retrieved from http://www.gallup.com/poll/166553/less-recommended-amount-sleep.aspx

[2]Harvard Medical School. *Insomnia Costing U.S. Workforce $63.2 Billion a Year, Researchers Estimate Insomnia appears prevalent in 23 percent of U.S. workers, higher in women.* Retrieved from https://hms.harvard.edu/news/insomnia-costing-us-workforce-632-billion-year-researchers-estimate-9-2-11

[3]Eric, Olson, Dr. *Diseases and Conditions Insomnia. Mayo Clinic.* Mayo Foundation for Medical Education and Research, 9 June 2015. Web.

[4]*How to Avoid Drowsy Driving.* Published by NHTSA's National Center for Statistics and Analysis 1 200 New Jersey Avenue SE., Washington, DC 20590 TRAFFIC SAFETY FACTS (2011): 1-3. Nhtsa.dot.gov. Mar. 2011. Web.

[5]Lineberry, Denise. *To Sleep or Not to Sleep?* NASA. N.p., 14 Apr. 2009. Web.

Chapter 4
[1]*Brain Basics: Understanding Sleep.* National Institute of Neurological Disorders and Stroke. Retrieved from https://www.ninds.nih.gov/Disorders/Patient-Caregiver-Education/Understanding-Sleep

[2]Kunz, Marie. *Caffeine And Anxiety,* 2013. Livestrong. Retrieved from http://www.livestrong.com/article/83671-caffeine-anxiety/

[3]McCarthy, Sky. *The Truth About Decaf Coffee,* 2014. Fox News Food & Drink. Retrieved from http://www.foxnews.com/food-drink/2014/08/25/truth-about-decaf-coffee.html

[4]Keefe III, John. H., D.C. *Sleep Problems,* 2016. Keefe Clinic. Retrieved from http://www.keefeclinic.com/wp/sleep-problems/

[5]Epsom Salt Council. *About Epsom Salt, The Science of Epsom Salt,* Retrieved from epsomsaltcouncil.org/about.

[6]Health.com. *Bedtime Behaviors that Work: 7 Habits That Will Prepare Your Body For Sleep,* Retrieved from http://www.health.com/health/condition-article/0,,20189095,00.html

[7]Fioravanti, Kayla. (2011) *The Art, Science and Business of Aromatherapy: Your Guide for Personal Aromatherapy and Entrepreneurship.* Franklin, TN. Selah Press. Print.

[8]Harvard Men's Health Watch. *Snoring Solutions,* Retrieved from http://www.health.harvard.edu/diseases-and-conditions/snoring-solutions

Chapter 5

http://abcnews.go.com/Health/american-heart-association-president-credits-cpr-saving-life/story?id=51990315

http://people.com/bodies/bob-harper-heart-attack-depression-suber-carb-diet-book-excerpt-exclusive/

[1]Chapman University. *America's Top Fears 2016*, Retrieved from https://blogs.chapman.edu/wilkinson/2016/10/11/americas-top-fears-2016/

[2]Paul, Marla. Northwestern. *Is Heart Disease Genetic Destiny or Lifestyle?* 2010 Retrieved from http://www.northwestern.edu/newscenter/stories/2010/11/heart-disease.html

[3]American Heart Association. *Stress and Heart Health.* Retrieved from http://www.heart.org/HEARTORG/HealthyLiving/StressManagement/HowDoesStressAffectYou/Stress-and-Heart-Health_UCM_437370_Article.jsp#.WL4TYIWcGt8

[4]Ace. *Exercise as a Cure For Fatigue and to Boost Energy Levels.* Retrieved from https://www.acefitness.org/acefit/fitness-programs-article/2742/acefit-workout-advice-and-exercise-tips/

[5]WebMD. *Exercise for Energy: Workouts That Work. Want to fight fatigue? Here's what kind of exercise--and how much--is best.* Retrieved from http://www.webmd.com/fitness-exercise/features/exercise-for-energy-workouts-that-work#1

[6]Karger. *Planner of Psychotherapy and Psychosomatics*, 2008, Retrieved from http://www.karger.com/PPS/
[7]Ace. *Exercise as a Cure For Fatigue and to Boost Energy Levels,* Retrieved from https://www.acefitness.org/acefit/fitness-programs-article/2742/acefit-workout-advice-and-exercise-tips/

[8]Mother Health Care. *Starting to Exercise: Senior Care and Disease Prevention*, Retrieved from https://clubalthea.com/2017/03/03/111421/

[9]Harvard Health Publications. Heartbeat. *5 of the Best Exercises You Can Ever Do,* Retrieved from http://www.health.harvard.edu/staying-healthy/5-of-the-best-exercises-you-can-ever-do

[10]Harvard Health Publications. Heartbeat. *Want To Live Longer And Better? Do Strength Training,* Retrieved from http://www.health.harvard.edu/staying-healthy/want-to-live-longer-and-better-strength-train

Chapter 6
[1]The Way Of The Seal, Think Like an Elite Warrior to Lead and Succeed, Mark Divine, Reader's Digest, New York, NY, page 80. 2013

Chapter 7
[1]*Adult Obesity Facts.* Center for Disease Control and Prevention. CDC, 21 Sept. 2015. Web.

[2-3]*Home Health 100 Million Dieters, $20 Billion: The Weight-Loss Industry by the Numbers.* ABC News. N.p., 8 May 2012. Web. [1]100 Million Dieters, $20 Billion: The Weight-Loss Industry by the Numbers

[4]Woolston, Chris, M.S. *What's Wrong With the American Diet?* Health Day. N.p., 20 Jan. 2016. Web.

[5]*Adult Obesity Facts.* Center for Disease Control and Prevention. CDC, 21 Sept. 2015. Web.

[6]Harvard T.H Chan. School of Public Health. *Economic Costs. Paying the Price for Those Extra Pounds.* Retrieved from https://www.hsph.harvard.edu/obesity-prevention-source/obesity-consequences/economic 2012

[7]Woolston, Chris, M.S. *What's Wrong With the American Diet?* Health Day. N.p., 20 Jan. 2016. Web.

[8]Olson, Samantha. *Refined Sugar vs. Saturated Fat: What's More Likely To Cause Coronary Heart Disease?* Medical Daily. N.p., 14 Jan. 2016. Web.

[9]Gunnars, Kris, BSc. *10 Disturbing Reasons Why Sugar Is Bad For You.* Authority Nutrition. N.p., n.d. Web. , BSc

[10]*Trans Fat Is Double Trouble for Your Heart Health.* Mayo Clinic. N.p., n.d. Web.

[11]*High Cholesterol.* Mayo Clinic. N.p., 9 Feb. 2016. Web.

[12]*Comfort Food.* Wikipedia. N.p., n.d. Web.

[13]Aldoori WH, Giovannucci EL, Rockett HR, Sampson L, Rimm EB, Willett WC. *A prospective study of dietary fiber types and symptomatic diverticular disease in men. J Nutr. 1998;128:714-9.*

[14]*Nutrition and Healthy Eating, Fiber: Daily Recommendations for Adults.* Mayo Clinic. N.p., 22 Sept. 2015. Web.

[15]Stobbe, Mike. *Skipping Breakfast May Increase Heart Attack Risk.* USA Today. N.p., 22 July 2013. Web.

[16]Covey, Alice, R.D., C.D. *How Dieting Can Be a Precursor to Eating Disorders.* BYU Idaho. N.p., n.d. Web.

[17]Selig, Meg. *Why Diets Don't Work...And What Does.* Psychology Today. N.p., 21 Oct. 2010. Web.

Health Habit Journal

The New Living Bible (NLT) Tyndale House Publishers. (2004). Holy Bible: New Living Translation. Wheaton, Ill: Tyndale House Publishers.

www.ingramcontent.com/pod-product-compliance
Lightning Source LLC
Chambersburg PA
CBHW071020280326

41935CB00011B/1430